IRRESIST[IBLY FIT]

How to Become a Spiritually Strong, Sexy, and Firm Woman
Everyone Admires and No One Can Resist

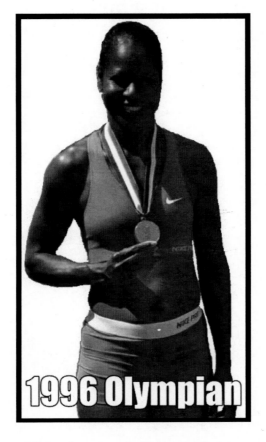

Being healthy and fit has been a priority in my life for many years now. I am always looking for new ways to not only challenge myself to greater health but also looking to bridge the gaps between health and fitness. Althea is one of the few fitness experts that I know (and I know quite a few) that has spent the time to investigate the proper foods and supplements that support a healthy mind, body, and spirit as well as stay on top of the latest exercise techniques. She understands the completeness of how to exercise for fitness and nourish the mind and spirit. If you want to get in shape, feel and look good, she is the one.
–Kashif (Six-time Grammy-nominated
R&B Music Legend, author, humanitarian)

IRRESISTIBLY FIT

How to Become a Spiritually Strong, Sexy and Firm Woman Everyone Admires and No One Can Resist

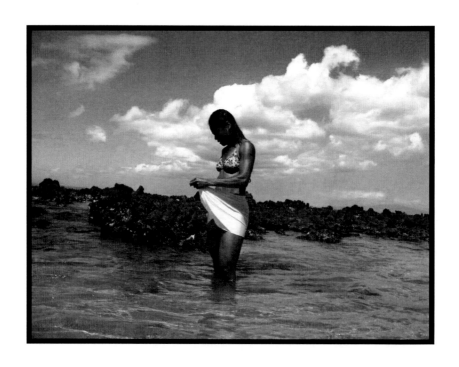

ALTHEA MOSES

#1 International – Bestselling
Author - Olympian
Speaker - Boss Lady of Fitness

IRRESISTIBLY FIT: How to Become a Spiritually Strong, Sexy, and Firm Woman Everyone Admires and No One Can Resist
Althea Moses, BA (UCLA), M.Ed (NU)

© 2013 © 2018 by Althea Moses. All rights reserved.

ISBN: 978-1-7321208-7-7
Library of Congress Control Number: 2018903546

© Photographs by Althea Moses

Photographs by Doug Duong and Althea Moses
Edited by Laurie Rosin and Candi Lawrence
Book formatting by bookclaw.com

Published in the United States by
AGM Group International Publishing
A division of
AGM Group International LLC
5250 W. Century Blvd., Suite 427
Los Angeles, CA 90045

Disclaimer: Irresistibly Fit provides information on a wide range of spiritual and fitness exercises, food science, health, and nutritional topics, and every effort has been made to ensure that the information is accurate. The advice and strategies contained herein may not be suitable for every situation or person. This book is not a substitute for expert spirituality, fitness, health, or nutritional advice, however, and you are advised to always consult a professional for specific information on personal spiritual, fitness, health, and nutritional matters. The authors, contributors, consultants, and publisher do not accept any legal responsibility for any personal injury or other damage or loss arising from any use or misuse of the information in this book.

If you find any typographical errors, please email the texts to be corrected. Thanks for your assistance.

Trademarks: ALTHEA, ALTHEA Fitness, and Circlemark are copyrighted in the U.S.A.

Moses, Althea.
Irresistibly Fit.

DEDICATION

This book is dedicated to my loving, talented, classy, courageous, intelligent, and beautiful mother, Candi Lawrence. Without you and God, I wouldn't be the woman I am.

Thanks for praying to God and raising us with God as our father.

Thanks for your courage to stand up to and leave daddy in 1980. You demonstrated that daddy's time was up, and you weren't afraid of traveling far away from your emotional and physical abuser.

Thanks for your unconditional love, support of my dreams, high standards, and choosing not to leave my four sisters and me behind when your mother returned to Belize for you.

Thanks for making incredible sacrifices for my sisters and me to live a decent life in Belize and better life in America—for being a good provider. I appreciate you for providing food for my sisters and me, while you went to bed hungry on many nights in Inglewood.

Thanks for expecting your daughters to get a high-school education and not becoming teenaged mothers. You're praised for rearing a three-time Olympian, college graduates, productive citizens, and successful entrepreneurs—Boss Ladies.

Thanks for modeling healthy living habits—not abusing your body with multiple men, drinking alcohol, smoking, and excess food.

Thanks for filing for my sisters and me to get our U.S. green cards immediately after your mother got her citizenship. Without you and our grandmother's assistance, we wouldn't have our U.S. citizenships, and would fear deportation like millions of immigrants in America today.

My beloved mother, I absolutely respect, appreciate, and love you!

SPECIAL THANKS TO MY FORMER COACHES

Starting at age 10, I had several great coaches on my athletic and Olympic journey. My former track star uncle, Luis, was my first track and bodybuilding coach. He invited me to run and lift weights with him.

Thanks to every coach for your time, dedication, finances, and health/fitness knowledge shared. You truly illustrated that you cared about my success in athletics and life. You set high standards, sought after special training/workouts just for me, and never wavered. You started me on my way to become one of the best athletes in Jr. Olympics and 1996 Olympics history.

MHS (Morningside High School) **track & field:** Ron Tatum, who taught me how to run long and fast, and coached me to a 3rd place finish in the California State meet and become the MHS record holder in the 800 meter run. I still hold the school record.

Johnny Estrada, who coached me in the pre-season to build up my endurance for regular season—and purchased my first pair of track spikes (shoes).

Darryl Taylor, who coached me in the triple-jump to become Morningside's first Jr. Olympic record-breaking-gold medalist and California State Champion in the triple-jump. He also helped me break many other high school meet records and set our school record too. I still hold the MHS triple-jump record.

MHS basketball: Mrs. Howard, who coached me on how to improve my basketball skills on the JV basketball team. Frank Scott, who invited me to play on his varsity team after my freshman JV season ended, and coached me as a forward for three and a half seasons—two with Lisa Leslie (former WBNA star and fellow Olympic Gold Medalist).

MHS cross-country: The coach who trained me to place 2nd in league finals, and run the CIF prelims—the one year (as a senior) I chose to run to improve my 800 meter times.

UCLA track & field: Bob Kersee, who trained me to improve my triple-jump skills and speed. Charles Yendork, who trained me to become a Silver Medalist in the PAC-10 Championships in

Triple-Jump, jump my personal best mark of 42 feet 8 ¾ inches, and earn my first paycheck as a professional track star. Bruin Brawn trainers for weight-training assistance.

Post-UCLA track & field: Greg Harper, who trained me (at USC) in the triple-jump to compete in the 1996 Olympic Games in Atlanta, GA, USA.

ACKNOWLEDGMENTS

Thank you Divine Creator of all people and things for: salvation through Jesus Christ, Holy Spirit, an amazing life of good health, love, peace, joy, prosperity, my strong spirit and firm-body temple. I honor you. Thanks for keeping, comforting, strengthening, healing, and prospering me—allowing your light to shine through me, and serving you through your people.

THANK YOU!

... My beautiful-intelligent grandmother (Egzine Gilharry-Lacy) for your love and courage, and coming to Belize to inspire my mother to bring my four sisters and me to Los Angeles—to take advantage of the opportunities America offers and live a safe and better life. Thanks for helping my mother and four sisters and me receive our U.S. green cards and citizenships! I miss you! I love you! (R.I.P.)

...Daddy for being a provider the first 10 years of my life (Belize). I appreciate you for building a house to reside, and providing food, and clothing. I miss you! I love you! (R.I.P.)

...My beloved-beautiful-talented family: Mother, Stephanie, Michelle, Paulette, and Lynette for your love and support of my endeavors (childhood to present). You're absolutely amazing! I love you!!!

...My former fiancé and beloved friend, Kashif Saleem—musical genius and humanitarian. Thanks for loving me with all your heart, your generosity, and inspiring me to be authentic without fear of ever losing anyone. Thanks for reviewing and supporting the first draft of my manuscript in 2014. I miss you! I love you! (R.I.P.)

...Every educator, counselor, coach, author, friend, and colleague who taught and assisted me.

...Joe Weider, for inventing the scientific principles of bodybuilding to build firm-body temples. (RIP)

...Robert Marshall (owner Huff Gym, Inglewood) for your amazing gym.

...City of Inglewood: Mayor Butts, Jr. and Council Members, Sabrina and Teresa (Parks & Rec.)

...Drs. Melvin and Sherrie Allen for coaching me how to build good personal/intimate relationships with men and be authentically me.

...My relatives, customers, clients, friends, fans, fellow athletes and Olympians, friends in the first Living Audacious Group Coaching for Women (LAGCFW) and The Projects Course for your encouragement, positive energies, love, business, and support.

...Linda and Diana (The Projects Course) for inspiring me to write a book and how to connect with my divine heart.

...Candi, Lynette, Donnette, Kamtoy, Subrina, Darryl, Tina, Alesia, Mike and Pam, Bashiri, Adrian, and Betty for showing me support/love as I grieved my loss in 2016. Kashif is smiling.

...Divine Heart, for helping me bring this book from my heart to reality—to share my knowledge, love of spirit and firm-body temple building.

...Michael and Scot for generous endorsements.

Write your name in the blank space if you've helped me: _____.

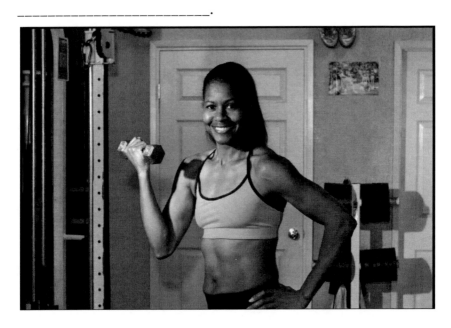

AFFIRM YOURSELF INTO SHAPE.TM

Table of Contents

INTRODUCTION

A legacy is born when something is created that enriches lives,
honors the past, and insures the future.
- McIver

Laid off from teaching elementary school, I looked for new
ways to earn income. I wanted to serve the world and make a
difference with my passion. I committed to and completed a couple
personal development programs—Living Audaciously Group
Coaching for Women and The Projects Course. Information and
support from both programs enlightened me on how to connect
with my heart and spirit through meditation.

In our first session, The Projects Course Director, Diana Vela,
said, "This is an awesome opportunity to bring something very
special to reality that has been waiting to be touched by you, and
brought to life from your divine, beautiful heart and soul."

I asked my divine heart and spirit, "What special thing do you
want me to bring to reality?" Meditating and listening to my heart
and spirit inspired me to write a mini-memoir and self-help book.
I'd teach how I became irresistibly fit despite a childhood with an
abusive father (Belize) and sexual molestation (Belize, Mexico, US),
and adulthood with abusive boyfriends and ex-husband.

You'll learn why I've been driven to be successful in
education, athletics, business, and not tolerate unloving- controlling-
abusive men.

Irresistibly Fit, teaches you about the benefits of having faith in
the Creator God, my early years growing up frighten with my
unloving-abusive father and abused mother (in Belize City), my
personal journey to the United States of America and three
Olympic Games, and hitting rock bottom after being blindsided by
betrayal of my trust. You'll also learn how techniques like *Althea
(mind/body/spirit)*, affirmations, Ho'oponopono (Hawaiian spiritual
practice), and prayers helped me look at my life as fixable, my heart
and spirit as repairable, and my firm-body temple as another source
of strength.

The use of these techniques helped me handle and triumph over decades of pain and suffering, and build my spirit and body temple rock solid.

Irresistibly Fit came from my heart and spirit to serve you, a whole, perfect emanation of our Creator God. With the Creator, I've cultivated my talents, skills, experiences, and passion to creatively express them as this book. Women and men of any age (who believe and work smart) can transform their spirit and body into a strong and firm-body temple.

You'll need to make a commitment to yourself, work hard and smart to live an active, healthy lifestyle. Also, you'll need discipline, consistent right actions, nutritional choices, my spiritual exercises, and cardiovascular and weight training. The weight-training routines were created (by me) for you to get results. My slogan: *Get Results With An Olympian's Touch.*

Although "exercise addiction" has gotten bad press, I'm so glad it's legal to exercise because I'm addicted, and I won't give it up.

This isn't just another health and fitness, or bodybuilding book. This is the first and only comprehensive mind, spirit, and firm-body temple training guide written by a three-time-track Olympian. It'll help you attain a strong spirit and firm-body temple by wedding the spiritual with the physical. It provides effective mind/spirit and body (cardio and weight-training) exercise routines to help heal you, and build your spirit and body temple into a rock-solid one. You'll be in tune with your mind, spirit, and body—and possess optimal health and wellness.

Since I started my health and fitness business, I've spoken to hundreds of women and men who have and are still suffering with bad memories, emotional pains, and lack effective ways to help them endure, overcome, and heal. They've tried exercising the body temple, but didn't feel better.

You can overcome your emotional pains and bad memories with spiritual exercises. I decided that I needed to share how I overcame pain and suffering to help billions of people. I feel pain and suffering test our faith, teach, purify, and strengthen our spirit.

Also, they show us when we feel we've lost everything and can't overcome pain and suffering, God and His love is always with us.

Love is giving someone the power to destroy you, but trusting them not to. – Anonymous

Several months after completing a personal development program, I felt my life was on hold because I was experiencing pain and suffering from betrayal. For a while, I was silent because I felt no one would believe I was betrayed. My faith and love was tested. I wanted my life to go on, but it was very difficult. I was inspired by Dr. Martin Luther King, Junior's quote, "Our life begins the day we stop being silent." I decided to stop being silent and move on with my life—be authentic.

I was also inspired to strengthen my spirit, feel better, and move forward with Ho'oponopono exercises. I did extensive research about it. This ancient practice strengthened my spirit and made me feel better the same day I started practicing it. I'll teach you how it helped me heal myself of all bad memories and the people and things involved--four phrases at a time.

With the mind/spirit exercises, you'll experience improved focus in every aspect of your life. You'll experience immediate results—with faith, open mind, and spirit. With the body (physical) exercises, your body will feel firmer in few weeks.

The illustrations and pictures show you how to work various muscle groups, effectively. The emphasis is on sculpting and strengthening your body into a firm-body temple that you'll be happy with when you look in the mirror. I want you to get the maximum benefit from your investment. With your great attitude, potential, discipline, and hard work, I believe you can achieve. I'm holding a space for you.

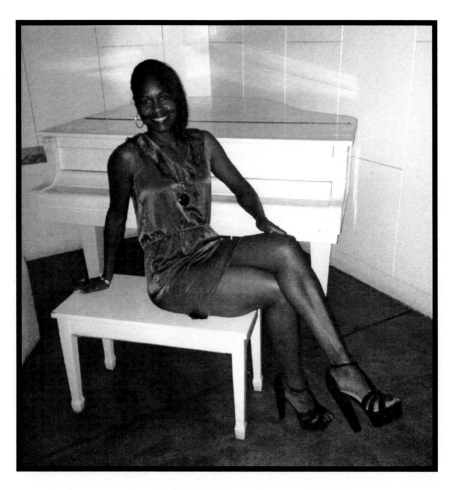

The journey is more important than the end result.

- John Wooden

CHAPTER 1

HOW I BUILT MY FIRM-BODY TEMPLE

As a child, I ran around and played hopscotch and other games with my peers. In junior and high school, I disliked my tall-skinny body, and big (size 10) feet. Along the way, I fell into track and field as a way to stay in shape after basketball season.

I enjoyed being in good shape from basketball training. The magic began the day I stepped onto the track and triple jump runway. I had no idea how great I'd become, how perfect my tall-skinny body temple and big feet would be for excellence. My high school coach certainly didn't know when we met. At some moment the realization dawned on us, and things took off from there.

I'm an excellent example of what commitment, tenacity, consistency, self-discipline, healthy eating and drinking, and cardiovascular and strength (weight) training can do for your body temple. For more than three decades, I've built and maintained my firm-body temple (a rock solid shrine, or sanctuary that's perfectly toned, fit, strong, shaped, sexy, and sensual) rock solid with mind, spirit, and body techniques.

Are you seeking effective ways to overcome your emotional pains and sufferings to live an authentic, rock solid life? Are you seeking to have a better, healthier body temple without stomach bulges, muffin tops, back creases, sagging arms, chest, and butt? Do your legs, thighs, hips, arms, and buttocks have cellulite and need firming up? Do you want to prevent or get rid of high blood pressure, high cholesterol, and diabetes diagnosis and medications? Then this book is right for you.

Irresistibly Fit teaches and illustrates techniques you'll need to transform your body temple into a firm, sexy, and sensual one. Almost two decades ago, I started referring to my body as a temple due to some Bible verses. They inspired me to treat my body as a temple.

I believe our body temple is a gift from the Divine God. People should do their best to take good care of their body temple, and honor God with it. I've been taking good care of my body temple to keep it looking and feeling younger—couple decades after competing in the 1996 Olympic Games.

My world-class running, triple-jumping, and weight training experiences have helped me become one of the best athletes in history. Now you'll benefit from my thirty-plus years of mind and spirit, Olympics and post Olympics (body) training skills, and basic nutritional knowledge. It'll help you build your spirit and body temple, feel great, and look younger than before. Everyone will admire you, and no one can resist you.

My journey to strengthen and maintain my mind, spirit, and body temple wasn't easy. I've had failures and successes, joyous and painful memories, and good people who loved, helped, and actions that hurt me. With faith in God and belief in myself, I've used my memories and mind/spirit, and body techniques to inspire and help me overcome all of my trials and disappointments, and achieve immediate success.

One of the techniques (exercise) that impacted my life is called *ALTHEA*. It's Greek for healing, healer, and wholesome. *ALTHEA*, is a combination of personal affirmations and exercise. I created this new mind, body, spiritual, love technique to heal, warm up, and exercise your body temple with your wholeness, power, sacred space, and love. Use it to exercise and heal your mind, body, and spirit daily.

Althea came to me as I was jogging and jumping in place to warm up for a workout. When the weather is cold outside, I exercise inside my home. I did what I usually do for warm up, but without my music playlist. As I was jogging, jumping, and raising my arms in front of my chest to above my head, I repeated the four Ho'oponopono phrases: "I'm sorry. Please forgive me. I love you. Thank you."

After fifteen minutes, I decided to do something different with my hands. I interlaced my fingers as if in prayer. Then I made a circle with my hands. I thought about the circle representing many things across the globe: wholeness, zero limits to my potential, unity, the sun that keeps us warm, sacred space, feminine power, and infinity.

I continued jumping and raising my circle hand gesture and arms over my head and repeated, "I love you," for about five minutes. I felt amazing and warmed up for my workout.

Then something astonishing happened. My mind and body transcended space, like I was floating on air. I felt wholesome, warm, powerful, protected, loved, and happier than before. In the midst of this experience, I smiled and decided that this simple fitness and spiritual technique could help and heal people globally, for generations.

I stopped and thought about a few things. The *Althea* technique can help change the world! People seeking love, to be loved, healing, good health, and wellbeing will benefit from it. When they exercise and repeat affirmations, they'll feel and look better in little time.

When you use my techniques, you'll be inspired and helped to overcome all trials and disappointments, and achieve success too. Do you believe that you can overcome and achieve whatever you strive to?

EARLY YEARS IN BELIZE CITY

What and who impacted me from childhood to adulthood?

I was birth from a very loving, strong, responsible, and resilient mother. She never gave up on her dreams about a better life for herself and her five daughters.

My mother was born and raised (Carol Gilharry) in Corozal Town in Belize. She's the eldest child of Egzine Gilharry and James Yearwood. My grandmother, Egzine, was of mixed race (East Indian father and African-descent mother), strict, and physically abusive. My grandfather, James, was nice—but an absentee father.

My grandmother had a difficult life in Corozal Town. When my mother was twelve years old, her mother abandoned her and eight siblings (four months to ten years old). She left them with her mother (Hazel Lawrence-Gilharry) in Corozal Town. My grandmother said her life was very difficult, so she abandoned all nine of her children and migrated to Los Angeles, California for a better life.

Unfortunately, after my grandmother left, my mother didn't have a better life in Corozal Town. Her childhood was very difficult because her grandmother emotionally and physically abused her. She expected my young mother to take care of six of her siblings. She slept on the floor of the tiny two-room house. When her baby brother cried at night, my great grandmother would wake her by beating her in her back with a large piece of wood. She was expected to take care of him.

My mother loved school. However, it was difficult because she was often sent to elementary school hungry. On her way to school, she'd stop by the local market's trash bin to retrieve half-rotten fruits for a meal. She cut off the rotten parts of fruits with a razor blade, and ate the edible parts for breakfast.

At age 13, my courageous mother ran away from her abusive grandmother. She moved to Belize City. She lived with one of her friend's family. While living there, she went to school. She started to have a stable life with people who didn't mistreat her.

While living at the friend's house, my mother met my father, Rudolph Moses. My father was sixteen years old. My mother was thirteen years old. He was born in Belize City, and still residing at home with his parents and siblings.

Before I was born, my parents were very young and exploring young adulthood. My father was clever, charming, dark, handsome, brave, and ambitious. He was tall (six feet, two inches) with a body temple built like "The Greatest" boxer of all time, Muhammad Ali. My mother was intelligent, charming, brave, ambitious, tiny, about five feet and three inches in height (ninety lb), light-skinned, and beautiful with long-black hair.

During their one-year courtship, he enjoyed being with my mother, his immediate family, socializing with male and lady friends, and riding his bicycle—his only form of transportation. The ladies chased him, and he chased them too. However, my mother was the one he took home to meet his mother, and the rest of his family.

My parents were alike in couple ways—responsible and liked each other.

My parents were different in other ways. She was ready to settle down with only him. He wasn't ready to settle down with only her. She wanted to migrate to Los Angeles to reconnect with her mother. My mother wanted to continue her education and pursue a fashion design career. He didn't want her to attend school or leave him. She wanted the best things in life. He wanted the basic things in life. He was a womanizer. She was committed to only him.

They started to have some problems because my mother didn't tolerate his womanizing, or hold her tongue. She was brave and authentic. She didn't have any problems expressing how she felt about my father's unacceptable behaviors. He disliked that about her.

When my mother was fourteen years old and my father was seventeen years old, something happened to them. They learned she was pregnant with me—their first child. My mother was very frightened.

My parents planned their lives together with their first child. As a result, my mother's life appeared to be getting better because my father chose to be responsible. He provided for her and their unborn child while still living with his parents.

In early 1970, I was born to two loving and responsible teenage parents, in Belize City Hospital. According to my mother, I was a healthy, beautiful baby girl with long arms and legs. She couldn't take her eyes off me. My parents were so grateful, and proud of their precious gift from God.

My father named me Althea—Greek name meaning healer, healing, and wholesome (health and wellbeing). My parents had no idea I'd become a high achiever in academics and athletics, or lover of health and wellbeing lifestyle.

My early days started on York Street in Belize City—in a one-room house with my mother. My father was seventeen and living at home with his parents. He rented the tiny house for us to reside until he was able to leave home. He showed he cared about my mother and me by providing safe shelter, food, and clothing.

According to my mother, he visited daily, and returned to his parent's home to sleep.

Unfortunately, a few months after I was born, my mother's life was becoming difficult again. One of my father's cousins informed her that my father named me after one of his mistresses. She asked my father if the allegation was true. He didn't deny it. He said his cousin talked too much!

My mother's track skills were on display! She didn't waste any time after hearing the disappointing news about how I got my name. She put on her track shoes and sprinted down to the Belize Registry Office to change my name. Unfortunately for her, the statute of limitations ran out to change my name.

My teen mother slowly walked back home feeling very disappointed. For months, she felt emotionally sick. Her life had gotten better and quickly worse due to my father's terrible choice. He was unapologetic about his behavior. My mother accepted the disappointment, and remained with him.

When I was six months old, my grandmother offered my fifteen-year old mother and me the opportunity of a lifetime. She wanted us to migrate to Los Angeles for a better life. My mother would be able to finish her grade school education, and pursue a fashion design career. Since age five, she had a dream to become a fashion designer.

My grandmother invited my mother to live with her and her new family in Los Angeles. She made travel arrangements for our departure in July 1970. My grandmother sent baby clothes and other items for our journey.

My mother was very excited about the journey to Los Angeles, and seeing her mother. She packed all of my diapers, clothing and other items in a new suitcase. Unfortunately, my father disapproved of her departure with their only child.

On a very hot and humid day before we departed, my father feared we wouldn't return to Belize, so he did something inconceivable inside our little home! My mother was holding me when she noticed a can of used engine oil in my father's hand. He was furious! He opened our new suitcase, and poured the entire can of engine oil onto my new diapers, clothing, and other baby items.

He grabbed me from her and held onto me. He told her that she could join her mother in Los Angeles, but without his daughter.

As my young and frightened mother wept, she thought long and hard about leaving her only child like her mother did (few years before). She thought about how I would suffer like she did as a child—how she'd suffer being away from me.

She decided to stay with my father. She said, "I couldn't leave my beautiful-baby girl." As a result of canceling her Los Angeles trip, my mother's life with my father got worse—a living hell.

The next few years of my life, both of my parents raised me in Belize City. They had three more daughters, together—Stephanie, Michelle, and Paulette. Would you believe my mother never allowed my father to name those daughters?

When I was two years old, my mother's teenage life continued to be difficult. Although my father was a good provider for our basic needs, he was controlling, insecure, and emotionally and physically abusive to my mother. He also continued to be a womanizer.

When I was about two years old, my father, 19, started another family with a much older woman who already had four children of her own. My mother and the other woman fought a lot—verbally and physically.

In 1972, both my mother and the other woman were pregnant for my father. My mother said that she was so embarrassed and ashamed—especially when she and the other pregnant woman passed by each other downtown Belize City.

Although my father betrayed my mother with the other woman, she remained with him because she was a sixteen-year old abandoned girl without family support, or a job. She was raising my one-year old sister and me. My mother felt that she was stuck between a rock and big mountain.

From age three to ten, I experienced a bittersweet childhood. I was raised in a strict home filled with my mother's love and nurturing. Our home was also filled with emotional, verbal, and physical abuse because my parents fought a lot. My mother said she fought to keep food on the table for her daughters. The issues of my father's alcoholic, jealous, and womanizing behaviors made it very difficult too.

As a result of the regular emotional, verbal and physical abuse I observed, I was always frighten and afraid when my father entered our home, and hearing my parents argue and physically fought. As a result, I vowed that I'd get an education, good job, and start a business in order to make my own money and not tolerate emotionally-physically abusive and controlling men like my mother and many other Belizean women did.

I was always happy whenever my father drove away from our home because he had a pattern of being absent for long periods of time. I often hoped he'd stay as long as possible, so my family and I would remain happy and safe.

When I was five years old, my family's life got better. At age 22, my father got a home loan to build his first house in Belize City. He designed and built it with his father's assistance. Although he had two families, he placed his first family (my mother, my three sisters, and me) in the new house.

My family and I were excited as we moved from the little-rented house on West Street to our new two-bedroom house on Benbow Street. It was a few houses away from my father's parents—Doris and Luther Moses.

My mother and my sisters, and I visited his parent's home daily because they were nice to us. They were raising several of daddy's nieces and nephews, so playtime at our grandparents' and our home was so much fun.

My mother became very close with my father's family. My grandmother treated her like her own daughter. She taught her how to cook, and be patient with my father's womanizing ways. My grandmother told my mother, "Look, I've been with his father for forty years and he just stop his womanizing." My mother responded, "I'm not waiting forty years for him to stop womanizing."

The next year in our new home, my mother gave birth to their fifth daughter--Lynette. Also, my father's mistress gave birth to twin boys—their third and fourth child.

21

Although my parents were intelligent and talented, they didn't complete elementary school. My mother got a little more education than my father, so she knew how to read, write, and spell well. On the other hand, my father didn't know how to write or spell as well. She helped him write for his business as needed.

In his twenties, my father went to a trade school to learn how to become an electrician. After he graduated, he became an electrician for the Belize Electricity Board and earned decent wages.

My mother loved sewing and fashion designing. She dreamed of becoming a fashion designer—designing and sewing fancy gowns. From basic knowledge she sewed women and children's clothing for school, work, and parties. She was such a talented seamstress that she had a regular clientele coming to our home.

In her twenties, my mother decided to attend a sewing school. Although she enjoyed sewing school, my father demanded that she drop out because one of my sisters wept often when she departed for class. Instead of offering to support her dream of education, my father demanded, "Stay home and mind (take care of) your f---ing kids." Although it broke her heart to dropout of school, she did so, and placed her fashion design dreams on hold.

As a result of being forced to place her vocational education on hold, my mother vowed and worked diligently to make sure that none of her daughters would never drop out of grade school, or be uneducated. She didn't want us to suffer like she did. I believed her, and I worked hard in school to get good grades.

Starting in Belize, she set high expectations for us. She repeatedly informed us to get a high school education. Education would allow us to make better choices than she did and have opportunities to experience a successful life—the opposite of her life as a child and young adult in Belize.

She was so serious about our education that she made sure she read to us, and we read to her. She also provided the necessary books and school tools. She made sure our homework was done and we studied for exams. She attended parent-teacher conferences, checked report cards, and disciplined us for bad grades. She repeatedly stated, "Get an education." It sounded like a broken record. Although her young life with my father was horrible, she never gave up on pushing and disciplining us to get an education!

My father was controlling. He didn't allow my mother to work. For a month, she earned thirty dollars at a sewing factory. He demanded, "Stay home! You're getting too much f--king big ideas!" When I was seven years old, my mother started a couple home businesses—mini-market and sewing. She needed income to support her five daughters because my father and his other woman had extended their family to four children—one girl and three boys. Fortunately for his other woman, my father supported her four children from a previous marriage. As a result, my father's income provided for shelter and food. My mother's income provided for clothing, footwear, school supplies, and medicine.

From about age seven, I was a very helpful and busy child. I didn't realize I was practicing entrepreneurship. I assisted my mother with the daily operations of her home businesses. I walked to and from the market and other stores to purchase food products for our home and the business. I cleaned our house, took orders, and completed sales. I even ran my own (play) store in our yard.

After all the work, I was still active. Sometimes I played with my cousins and friends in the neighborhood. We went walking, running, bike riding, played hopscotch and softball, and jump roping.

Our home was usually warm and loving until my father showed up—after staying out one to few nights per week. My mother wanted him to change his ways and stay home with us. But he was selfish and did whatever he wanted.

He told her what she could and couldn't do. She couldn't take us to the beach, straighten (perm) her hair, stay out late, have friends, or her family members visit, and question him about his relationship with other women, and sleeping elsewhere at night. When she did any of these, he'd grab, slap, push, slam, or punch her. Then a fight starts because my mother fought back until she couldn't take the pain anymore.

After the fights, my father would leave for days. Then my sisters and I helped her wipe blood and tears of pain from her beautiful-abused face. I often wished and prayed that I was older to stop him from abusing my mother.

Although my father was tall, dark, and handsome, he was very insecure. He hated when his male cousins and friends stated, "You have a beautiful woman." During Christmas holidays, he'd invite his male friends to dinner and drinks. When anyone commented about his woman being beautiful, he became furious. This behavior caused her to leave, and visit my grandparents until his male friends left.

My father was insanely jealous! Once, he told my mother that he'd disfigure her pretty face, so that no man would want her. My mother wasn't one to hold her tongue, so she responded, "It's the hole between my legs that men want." He got furious! He slapped her so hard, she said that she saw stars!

The verbal and physical abuse at the hands of my father towards my mother was consistent in our household. My mother often fought back. Many times, she got tired and frustrated, and left him. She took us to our paternal-grandparents' home, and left for a little time to figure out what to do next. She took care of us in the daytime, but departed in the evening. Then my father would find her and physically force her to return home.

When I was eight years old (1978), my mother got angry about my father's womanizing, controlling, and abusive behaviors that came with daily shame and embarrassment. With bravery and courage, she (23) decided that she wouldn't tolerate it anymore.

One night, my mother asked God for help and got a rapid response. She asked my father, "What should I do for you to leave me? He replied angrily, "You go and fight that woman one more time and I'll leave you!"

The following day, my fed up and courageous mother took my father's advice. She fought my father's mistress in public. My mother knew that she'd be in grave danger.

Later that evening, my mother packed a small bag and informed us that we were going to stay with her sister in Belize City. I was excited to hear that because they were a happy family that I'd never seen fighting.

It wasn't long before my father showed up at my aunt's home—drunk, furious, and demanding. It was nighttime. Both families had just prepared to go to sleep before my uncle left his home. Before leaving, he told my mother and aunt not to open the door until he returned.

Minutes after my uncle left, there was a knock at the front door. My mother thought it was my uncle, so she opened it. She and I were shocked to see my father! My stomach felt sick and my little heart stopped for a moment. I knew what would happen next.

He stood at the front door, grabbed her nightgown with her in it, and demanded that she get her things to return home. But my mother didn't want to return because she was unhappy and unsafe there. My sisters and I felt unsafe too.

My father demanded, "Let's go home!" She replied, "No!" He quickly raised his hand and punched her in her mouth, like a boxer punched by Muhammad Ali. My aunt, sisters, and I screamed as we watched my mother's ninety-pound body fall to the floor—in pain while holding her bloodied mouth. I was shocked and frightened! I wanted to hurt him back, but I was afraid! My aunt said my father pulled out a long screwdriver from his pocket, but her boyfriend took it away from him. I often cry and thank God for saving my mother from being stabbed to death in front of my sisters and me.

My abused mother was wailing. My aunt, sisters, and I were screaming and crying. I felt helpless as my father grabbed and pulled my mother's tiny body like she was a rag doll. Her face was disfigured. Two of her front teeth hung from her bloodied-upper gum. Tears of pain, and saliva and blood ran down her beautiful face and nightgown.

My father was determined to take us back home, so he pulled my mother's tiny body and pushed her into the front seat of his station wagon. My sisters and I got into the backseat as we cried and felt compassion for our mother. She was in agony. There was nothing we could do. My father was so coldhearted! He did nothing to ease her pain.

That night, my father demonstrated that he was a heartless tyrant. Although my mother needed medical attention, he drove us home instead of to a hospital.

When we arrived home, he sat on our front stairs. He watched my mother take our clothes from the car. Then to further embarrass her, he shouted, "I want the whole f--king neighborhood to see how I disfigured her pretty face!" All I could do was look at my mother and feel empathy for the pain and embarrassment she was experiencing. I was so angry that I wanted to kill my father.

My father didn't apologize or comfort my mother. He fell asleep with his hand holding her down on the bed. For sometime, my mother moaned and wailed because her mouth was in excruciating pain. Two-front teeth still hung from her gum. My father refused to take her to the dentist. I wondered how a man could treat the mother of his children so cruel.

An hour later, my father drove my mother to a dentist because she got up to walk there in her bloodied nightgown. The dentist extracted her two-front teeth.

Couple hours after my parents returned from the dentist, my mother decided that she didn't want to live with my father. Before dawn, she left our home and ran to a friend's house in her bloodied nightgown. My father didn't know where she was.

Few days later, my mother heard that my father wanted her to come home. She told my paternal grandmother to inform my father that she was willing to return under two conditions—he must move out of the house and have no more sex with her. Initially, he disagreed with her conditions. After talking with his mother, he agreed. My mother said that she returned home to take care of her five daughters because she didn't want my grandmother, or my father's other woman to take care of us.

My father moved out of our home. He lived with his other family. For the next eighteen months, he provided a house and money for food. Once a week, he visited my sisters and me. Our home was somewhat peaceful and fun because there were less arguments. I was fearful and unhappy whenever he visited.

My mother decided that she had to leave Belize to protect herself and five daughters from our father. This time, she knew that she had to go far away from Belize City.

My mother contacted her mother, who resided in Los Angeles. She explained the emotional and physical abuses that she was experiencing, and why she believed that my father was going to kill her. My mother said, "If you don't help me get away from my abuser, you'll come to bury me!"

I kept thinking how my father had finally disfigured my mother's beautiful face—just as he had threatened to keep men from looking at her. Her beautiful smile was gone because there was a large gap in her mouth. I hoped that my mother could take us someplace far away, so my father could never abuse her again—or kill her.

My grandmother offered my mother to travel with my sisters and me to Los Angeles—far away from my father. This time, my mother told my father that we were going for summer vacation. We were so excited when he agreed to let us go!

Days later, my father changed his mind about us leaving for vacation. My mother listened to my grandmother's advice and stopped arguing with him. She told my father, "Okay, we're not going." However, her mind, hands, and feet continued planning.

My mother made sure that her mouth was gapless while traveling. She purchased a partial to replace the two teeth that my father had punched out of her mouth.

My mother did some important things before leaving my father. First, she prevented my sisters and me from informing anyone about our trip to Los Angeles. Then she saved money for the costs of the five-day journey. She prayed for protection, guidance, and success daily.

Before we left Belize, my mother didn't want my father's family and our neighbors to know that she was leaving forever. She stopped all communication with her best friend, neighbors, and my father's family. She confided in only one good friend who agreed to keep her secret, store our packed luggage, school-transfers and other legal documents.

In spite of the last beating my mother, 25, got from my father, 28, while she planned to leave him, the Plan remained in progress. She said, "I wanted to die with the rest of my teeth in my mouth."

27

In 1978, the second Get-Away Plan (Plan) began. It wasn't like the first plan when I was six-months old. My mother planned with a good friend. She gave the friend luggage filled with two pieces of clothes for each of us. She was instructed to deliver the luggage to the bus terminal at eleven in the morning—an hour before the bus was scheduled to depart.

The Plan was similar to the Underground Railroad (during slavery times) in the USA. In the middle of the night, one of my uncles knocked on our door and informed my mother that we'd depart the following morning.

My mother, and my sisters and I were excited about going far away from our father, but the excitement was overshadowed by our nervousness. My mother stated, "If your father knew that I planned to leave him the following morning, he probably would've killed me." I believed her.

About an hour after my uncle left, my mother placed me on watch duty with the lights off. She told me to sit at the window to see when my father drove up to our home.

Minutes later, I couldn't believe what I saw—my father's car was turning the corner. I felt my little heart jump out of my chest and hit the floor! Immediately I ran into the kitchen with my heart trailing on the floor. I yelled to my mother, "He's coming!" She told my sisters and me to lie down on the floor, and to pretend like we were sleeping. We did so. Then she ran to the bedroom with my baby sister, closed the door, and pretended like they were sleeping.

In the unlit house, my heart was beating the walls of my tiny-overworked chest. For a short time, I watched my father walk by my sisters and me quietly. He looked at us as we pretended to sleep on the living-room floor. Then he walked to my mother's bedroom, opened the door, looked in briefly, and closed it. Then he left. All of us were relieved, but still nervous.

Minutes later, my mother ran to her friend's house to inform her to meet us at the bus terminal in the morning.

In the morning, my sisters and mother, and I walked from our home with uncombed hair, dirtied clothes, and barefooted. My mother asked us dress this way in order not to bring attention to our secret departure.

In the bus terminal's restroom, my mother, her sister (Laverne), and her friend helped my sisters and me change into our new clothes and sandals. Then they combed our hair.

We got settled and sat quietly as we waited for the bus to depart. I looked through the bus window and thought about the unknown place (Belizeans call "States") that we were traveling to. I wondered if it was better than Belize. Also, I thought about how our father would never physically and emotionally abuse my mother again.

Then the bus started moving out of the terminal. I wept as thoughts of not seeing my other grandparents, aunts, uncles, cousins, and friends anymore. My mother hugged me and said everything is going to be better for us.

About two days on our bus journey, we came to a Mexican checkpoint. The bus was filled with passengers. A border-patrol agent entered the bus. He walked towards my mother. She was frightened. We were the only ones escorted off the bus and taken to a small room for questioning. The agent asked, "Where are you going?" My mother said, "I have a Mexican visa. We're going on vacation to Acapulco." The border-patrol agent responded, "I'm not stupid. We know a lot of you pass through here to go to California." The agent demanded that my mother pay twenty-five dollars (US) per person in order to return to the bus. She paid it.

We rode on the next bus through Mexico to the Mexico/US border. But it wasn't without incident. For couple hours, we waited for another bus in front of the terminal. My mother became frightened because the last bus didn't arrive as scheduled, and Immigration Officers were known for racial profiling. Then God sent an angel (a taxi driver) to save us from Mexican Immigration Officers. The taxi driver informed my mother that the officers would pick us up, take us to the immigration holding area, and send us back to Belize. My mother pleaded with him to help us not get arrested. We got into his taxicab and he drove us to his home.

For the next few days, we stayed with the taxicab-driver, his wife, and toddler. They allowed us to stay in one of their bedrooms and provided food and water too. While inside the bedroom, I was sexually molested. I didn't inform my mother because I didn't want to get in trouble with my molester. They told me not to tell or else...

My mother communicated (by telephone) with a family member in Los Angeles. They worked out the details of the journey to the Arizona border and Los Angeles.

CROSSING THE BORDER AND LIFE IN LOS ANGELES

After six days in Mexico, another good-hearted person drove us across the border into the United States of America. The Get-Away Plan was successful! Upon arrival, we thanked God for protection and opening the doors to come to America.

My family and I embraced each other as we wept with relief and joy. We thanked God for blessing us on our long-challenging journey to the United States of America. We celebrated freedom from my abusive father, and started a new and better way of living in my grandparent's home in Los Angeles.

That same summer, I was enrolled in a fifth-grade class at West Athens Elementary School. Schoolwork wasn't difficult for me, but adjusting to my new school environment was challenging. Some students teased me about my used clothing, supermarket footwear, and Belizean language/accent.

For a few months, I was teased and bullied by couple classmates. Everyday in class, a boy sat behind me and pulled my braids. I told him to stop. One day I reached my limit with the boy pulling my braid, so I turned around and closed my eyes. Then I grabbed and launched him across the desk. As for the girl, she pushed me on our way home. I grabbed her and we fought. Then we became best friends.

Sometimes my mother, sisters, and I were mistreated at my grandparent's house. My grandmother abandoned nine kids in Belize. Then she had three young kids (11, 9, and 7) with her African-American husband. The house was full. They tried adjusting to living with nine immigrants—their family. We tried adjusting to them too. Sometimes we had nice times, but other times, my uncles and aunts mistreated us. Sometimes we were locked out of the house for hours. Again, I was sexually molested in our house. I didn' t inform anyone due to fear of harm to my mother and me.

My family and I were uncomfortable and frightened as we resided at my grandmother' s house. We slept on their bedroom and living room floors. After school, my sisters and I had to wait in the front of the house, or in the backyard until my mother returned from working in the sewing factories. We kept ourselves busy at the local middle school, or our grandparent' s front yard. As a result, I dreamed and hoped for a home of our own.

Summer 1981, my dreams and hopes of residing in a house with our own family bedrooms became reality. My mother met a kind and generous man. He loved her and cherished her feelings. He listened to her cries to move out of my grandparent' s house before the summer ended. He offered to rent a house for all of us to reside. My mother accepted his offer and we started plans to move.

EARLY YEARS IN INGLEWOOD

Before I started sixth grade, our family moved into a small house near the Forum arena in Inglewood, California. We were excited to reside in a home without any family mistreatment or sexual molestation. After sleeping on the floor for a year, it felt so good to sleep in a bed again!

My mother worked hard for us! She said, "You girls gave me strength to get up and go to work." I recall my sisters and I running to hug her as she walked off the RTD bus on Crenshaw/108th Street. She said, "Although I was exhausted, you girls brought so much joy to me--every evening I walked off the buses."

In Inglewood, I helped my mother raise my sisters. I was the babysitter while she was at work. Also, I had an active lifestyle from sixth to eighth grade. I often walked, ran, and rode my bicycle. At age ten, I started playing basketball and performing weight lifting with one of my uncles. He was a member of his high school's cross-country and track teams.

While in sixth grade and junior high school, I practiced running and weight training with my uncle. He earned a college-track scholarship, so I was inspired to earn one too. I felt it was an excellent resource to get a free-college education.

My freshman year, I attended Morningside High School. It was a big school. It was known for its successful academic and athletic students, amazing teachers, athletic coaches, and sports teams. My best friend, Kamtoy, was there too, so I felt comfortable.

This first year was busy and challenging as I adjusted to my new environment, and started playing junior and varsity basketball.

After basketball season ended in March, I was in good shape and had a lot of time on my hand. However, I wasn't excited about going home after school because there wasn't much to do, and my neighborhood was noisy and challenging with gang activities. Also, I didn't want to be idle or get out of shape. Importantly, I felt I needed to continue practicing hard in order to reach my goals—use my intelligence and athletic abilities to earn a full-college scholarship, move out of the "ghetto" or urban neighborhood, and experience a better life than my parents did.

To reach my goals, I decided to join the track team. I heard that Ron Tatum was the head track coach and one of the best running coaches in the area. Also, I heard that outdoor season was already underway and he was a tough coach. Even so, during my Physical Education period, I got dressed for track practice and planned to meet him on the track.

The magic began the day I set foot onto the large-dirt track. My future track coach and I had no idea how great I'd be, how perfect my tall-skinny body with big feet would be for excellence. I felt nervous as I walked toward Coach Tatum. Then I got distracted. My eyes got a glimpse of some handsome-male athletes whose bodies were muscled-toned—just the way I enjoyed seeing them. At that moment, I felt I had to work hard to make the track team.

I felt nervous as I got closer to Coach Tatum. I felt more nervous as my eyes set upon the handsome-muscle-toned man with mustache and low-neat afro. He was tall and appeared to be a tough coach. I walked over and introduced myself to him.

I stated, "I just finished my first varsity basketball season. I'm interested in joining the track team. How do I get started?"

Coach Tatum welcomed me with a friendly smile and directed me to the large circle of athletes as they were warming up to start practice. Some senior athletes lead the stretching routine from the middle of the circle. That day, I decided that I'd become one of the leaders in that circle.

After assessing my running ability, Coach Tatum told me to run the 800 m event. During and after running that event, I was exhausted! Then he told me to perform the triple-jump (run, hop, step, and long jump) on an asphalt runway and into pit with a low amount of sand. This was difficult to perform, but I didn't quit. Since I'd never performed the triple-jump event, I felt awkward. I wondered if I'd ever get better.

Coach Tatum was dedicated to having all his athletes becoming champions and earning track scholarships, so he had some other talented coaches to teach us too. During my freshman year, Mrs. Howard coached the jumping events and Johnny Estrada coached the hurdling events.

As the track season progressed, I believed that Coach Tatum could help me become a champion. I listened to him and did whatever he suggested. He taught me correct running and weight lifting techniques, and how to run faster too. I practiced on and off the track. I watched what I ate and drank—especially before track practice and meet days. Also, I got as much rest as I could.

Our practices felt like mini-track meets because most athletes ran every race very fast. Monday through Friday, we performed grueling timed workouts that hurt badly—especially on Mondays! For example, the painful thousand breakdowns (1,000 m, 800 m, 600, 400 m, 200 m, 150 m) were exhausting. We were expected to run those races within a certain time or we would have to rerun them. I made up my mind to run the times, so I didn't rerun any races.

After the running workouts, I performed grueling triple-jump workouts on the grass, runway, and into the sand pit. I was on the track for more than two hours and in the weight room for about an hour—four times a week. As a result, I was exhausted! However, I remembered my goals and often affirmed that working hard would pay off.

The day before my first league meet, I was elated because I made the varsity team. I received my first varsity-track uniform. I couldn't wait to tell my mother, so I ran home and waited for her to arrive from work. She was excited for me. My mother congratulated me with a loving hug and stated her usual phrase, "Go after your goals and dreams. I believe you can do it."

Did I have support of my family at my track meets? My mother wasn't always there. However, that didn't bother me. I knew that my mother (a single mother) loved me and supported my dreams. When she had it, she gave me five dollars for lunch before I left for track meets. She provided a safe-loving home environment with the basics for me to strive for my goals. Also, I understood that she wasn't there often because she worked hard in the Los Angeles sewing factories, and needed to take care of my four younger sisters—she needed to rest her hardworking body.

My first league meet was scary because a lot of athletes appeared to be faster and stronger than me. I was nervous as I stood in my lane to run the 800 m race. Inside of my stomach felt like butterflies were dancing. As soon as the gunshot sounded, I ran ahead of all of the other girls for both laps around the track. I had some competition, but I ran fast enough to win the race. I was exhausted, but relieved and happy it was done!

After I recovered from running, I walked over to perform the triple-jump event. I ran down the runway, hopped, stepped, and long jumped into the sand pit. The meet attendant measured my distance and informed me that I was now leading the competition with a mark of 30-plus feet. I didn't have anything to compare my mark to, so I wasn't excited. Coach Howard and some of my teammates got excited and congratulated me with hand slapping, kind words, and smiles because the mark surprised them. The other school's athletes had the look of worry on their faces, so I got excited and thought that I must be really good at jumping.

This was one of the first times I felt accomplished and valuable to our track team. After several jumps, I won the competition. I was happy to experience the winning feeling at my first track meet!

Throughout the rest of the season, I ran the 800 m race faster and triple-jumped farther. I kept winning my running and jumping events at the other league meets.

Then I competed in the final league meet of the season— Pioneer League Championships. I felt confident that I'd win my first gold, silver, or bronze medals because I was stronger and faster and I already beat the same athletes.

At league finals, I believed that I'd win the gold medal in the 800 m run. I won it. I believed I'd win a medal in the triple-jump. I did. At the time, I didn't know what it meant, but winning qualified me for a trip to the CIF Section preliminary meet (prelims).

I was elated about winning my first pair of track and field medals, but nervous about competing in the CIF meet because the competition was going to be tougher than at our league meets. But Coach Tatum assured me that I was ready to compete with some of the best athletes in southern California. I believed him.

The next weekend, our school bus drove into the huge parking lot at Valencia High School. My eyes got big and I felt nervous! This was the day that I got my first introduction to serious track and field competition. Thousands of athletes and coaches were preparing for the all-day track meet. This was the meet to qualify for the next week's CIF section finals at Cerritos College.

As I walked passed the track, I felt like butterflies were dancing in my stomach again. I imagined crossing the finish line first and jumping the farthest. I felt the tension from many athletes. I knew that I had to run faster and jump farther to qualify for the following week's final championship meet—my next opportunity to ride the bus and win more medals. I affirmed that I'd do my best.

The gunshot sounded. I ran my best 800 m time and jumped my best triple-jump mark of the season, but I didn't qualify to compete in the CIF finals meet. Although, I was grateful, my heart was broken.

Afterwards, Coach Tatum congratulated me for performing my best in both events. I wept silently in the girl's restroom. I replayed the race in my head many times. I wondered what I could've done better to win it. Then I affirmed that I'd be a CIF champion the next year.

My first track season concluded with a gold medal and personal bests in the 800 meter run (2 minutes and 25 seconds) and triple-jump (35 feet and 3 inches). I was happy with my track achievements, but not content.

At the annual, track and field banquet, many of my senior-class teammates received trophies for their performances. Before it ended, I got an amazing surprise. I was awarded the "Workhorse" trophy. I was happy and grateful for their recognition. That night I knew there was something special about me—my coaches recognized it.

I thought about winning more medals and trophies, breaking our school records, winning at the CIF finals and State meet, the scholarship, and becoming an Olympian.

My sophomore year was the start of the best years of my track career because I became a school-wide and local track star. I got a new triple-jump coach. I learned how to run with correct technique and paced myself better. My track skills improved immensely and my event marks were phenomenal! I started wearing my signature track gear—red headband and ponytail hairstyle. Kamtoy moved, so I had best friends on the track team--Antonio and Ray. I was on my way to becoming a state champion and an Olympian.

Coach Tatum wanted me to be the best 800 m runner in the world. His new approach to training me was elevated to another level than the prior year. He challenged me and I challenged myself every time I set foot on the track.

In practice, Coach Tatum made me run with the middle distance varsity boys. It was very difficult, but I was determined to do what it'd take to become a track and field champion. I worked very hard to stay close and beat them to the line too. One day I came close to beating John Mason--one of the junior-class boys. After the race, he stated that I scared him. I smiled and set out to beat him every time we raced. He never allowed me the pleasure of beating him.

Coach Tatum wanted me to be the best triple jumper in the world. My sophomore year, he hired Darryl Taylor—a UCLA triple-jump alumni and 1988 Olympic hopeful. After meeting Coach Taylor, I realized we had some things in common—he was kind, a dreamer, driven to succeed, and enjoyed the triple-jump event. Those things made me feel comfortable as we worked together. I believed that he could help me become a champion, so I listened and did whatever he suggested.

During practice, Coach Taylor made me perform the triple-jump repeatedly—sometimes until the sun went down. This happened so often that some teammates joked, "Your coach trains you until the cows come out!" I remembered Coach Taylor stating, "Give me one more good one." One more became three and four more.

During the season, I bounded on the grass for fifty-plus meters. I hopped, stepped, and long jumped on the runway and into the sand pit—ten to fifty times. Then I hopped over three to six hurdles at a time--boxes too. After all of that, I had to run my grueling 800 m workout and weight room training. After every practice, I was exhausted. But I believed that I had to do the hard work to win races and jumps, and qualify for a full track scholarship.

As my sophomore track season progressed, Coach Taylor and I spent a lot of time on and off the track and runway. My family and I grew to know him well. My mother and I trusted Coach Taylor. She said, "I felt good about Darryl. I had no doubt about him caring for and protecting you." I knew Darryl's girlfriend, friends, and family. I felt like I was his little sister. His family became my extended family. To this day his mother calls me "my baby."

I knew Coach Taylor truly cared about his athletes because he often asked after jumping, "How did that feel?" He wanted us to raise our awareness so we could be in tune with our body. "You must assess where you are and make adjustments on the runway," he explained. Today, I ask my health and fitness clients the same question during our sessions--for the same reason.

Coach Taylor wanted me to be the best 800 m runner and triple-jumper in the world. Sometimes he ran the last 100 meters of some of my strenuous 800 m workouts with me. It helped me run faster when I was very tired at the end of races.

To improve my jumping technique, Coach Taylor trained me with other college and high school athletes. I was usually the only girl at those practices, so I worked hard to scare and beat the boys. I was happy when he took me to triple-jump and weight train with some world-class triple-jumpers at UCLA and Mount SAC, like Milan Tiff and Ray Dupree.

Coach Tatum cared about me too. He took his top athletes to local invitational track meets on the weekends. Those meets were so much fun because there were thousands of talented athletes, food, hot weather, picnic gear, and more medals to win.

This second track season, I worked harder on and off the track. I became stronger and faster. I learned how to pace myself in the 800 meter run. I wasn't as tired as the year before. Also, I learned the techniques to triple-jump farther.

I learned that Coach Tatum's athletes didn't get spring break week to rest or have fun traveling with family. We traveled with him and his team of coaches. It wasn't for our pleasure. We went to a local dirt hill and ran up and down. We pulled car tires on the grass and ran on the track. Afterwards, we weight trained and performed abdominal exercises. Those spring practices were grueling, but we got stronger and faster to excel at what we called "The Big Meets"— Mount SAC, League and CIF finals, Masters, and the ultimate California State meet.

Towards the end of my sophomore track season I was excited and grateful. I was jumping farther and running faster. I won Pioneer League-gold medals in the 800 meter run (2 min. 22 sec.), triple-jump (37 ft. 6 in.), and long-jump (16 ft. 5 in.). As a result, I became a school-wide and local track star. I felt accomplished when I started seeing my name and marks in the sports section of local newspapers—Los Angeles Times and Wave.

The following week, I returned to the CIF Preliminary (prelims) meet. When I walked onto the track to run the 800 m race, I looked into the crowded stands and saw some of my teammates and coaches. My stomach felt like the butterflies were dancing inside again. When the gun sounded, I ran the first curve fast and then stayed with the group of runners until the last straightaway.

When I heard the huge crowd cheering and yelling, I shifted my speed and ran fast enough to finish in the top three. I was elated and exhausted—my run was much better than the prior year. I knew that I qualified for next week's finals in Cerritos. When I saw my name on the 800 meter Qualifier's document, I jumped with joy and clapping with happy tears.

The next week, I walked into Cerritos College's huge sports stadium with nervousness, pride, and joy. The track was blue and the stadium and audience reminded me of the one I saw at the 1984 Olympic Games in Los Angeles—couple years prior. It was electrifying!

As I walked onto the track to run the 800 m race, it felt like butterflies were dancing inside my stomach again. When the announcer introduced me by name, I looked into the crowded stands for Coach Tatum, but I didn't see him. I smiled and waved. The crowd cheered loudly. Then my eyes filled with tears as I thought about how Coach Tatum taught me to become a championship runner—as a sophomore I was one of the top CIF Division 2A - 800 m runners.

I heard the meet starter say, "On your mark. Get set." Then the gun sounded. I ran the first curve fast and stayed with the group of runners for the first lap and a half. Then I increased my speed as I set my eyes on the last one hundred straightaway. There were two girls close to me. They were running as fast as me. I tried to run faster as I looked at the tape at the finish line. However, my body felt like a zoo of animals jumped onto my back. I felt like I was running in slow motion and couldn't run any faster!

The race was very close. I heard the crowd get louder. I wanted to run faster, but I felt like I ran out of gas. I kept pushing myself to pass the girl running almost next to me. I tried to run past her, but she wasn't slowing down. As we got closer to the finish line, she leaned across it before I did. I smiled at the winner and said, "Good run." My tears flooded my eyes as I walked off the track and breathed rapidly.

I got the silver medal instead of the gold I hoped for. However, I was happy to earn my first medal at the CIF Finals. I walked off the track, rested my hands on my knees to recover. I felt like collapsing on the field like many other girls did. Instead, I looked up at the large scoreboard. I saw the winner and my name and running times—2:15.03 and 2:15.04. My tears flood my eyes again and I smiled with gratitude. I said aloud, "Wow! I almost won my first CIF gold medal."

I remember jumping with excitement when I realized how close I came to winning. My tears rolled down my face as I thought about what I had accomplished in two years. I ran (2:15.04) two minutes and fifteen seconds. That's ten seconds faster than I did the previous (freshman) year. After that race, I believed I had the talent to compete in the State Meet and Olympics.

I was proud that I reached couple of my personal-track goals: broke our school record by one second and I got my first CIF finals medal. Additionally, I qualified to run the 800 m event at the CIF Masters meet the following week. I felt excited! Masters is the track meet that nine athletes in each event will compete to qualify for the last high school track meet of the year—The California State Track and Field meet. This is where each athlete demonstrates they're the best (in the state) in their event(s) and medals placed around their neck, just like at the Olympics.

After the race, I experienced my first medal presentation on an Olympic-styled platform in the center of the stadium. The first place medalist stood on a higher platform than me. The third place medalist stood slightly lower than me. Our names, school's name, and times were announced as we stood on the platform. I held my silver medal and glanced over at the gold medal I wanted. My heart was still elated! Tears of joy flooded my eyes. I smiled and waved to the cheering crowds. The official photographer took our pictures. This was the ultimate experience of champions—recognition of our hard work, commitment, and dedication. I believed that experience was the start of many leading up to the Olympic Games.

When I returned to our team's location in the warm up area of the stadium, my coaches, teammates, and friends congratulated me with hugs, high fives, and verbal praises—"Way to go, Althea!" I felt like a star.

Later on, I recovered from the 800 m race and prepared to compete in the triple-jump. I felt nervous because the triple-jumpers looked like they were skillful and ready to jump far. I was ready to jump farther than before.

As I walked onto the blue-triple-jump runway, I felt like butterflies were dancing inside my stomach again. It was time for introductions before our event began. All of the jumpers and I stood in a line (on the runway). We faced the track fans. They cheered loudly. When the announcer said my name, I looked into the crowded stands, smiled, and waved. I became emotional. My tears flooded my eyes and my spirit moved. I felt nervous.

Like the 800 meter run, the competition was fierce. The top four jumpers were executing well. Our marks were within couple inches of each other. After completing all six jumps, I placed third with a mark of 37 feet 6 3/4 inches—a personal record (P.R.). My mark was less than two inches of the first and second place marks. I felt happy that I won my second CIF medal (bronze) and was returning to the presentation platform. My third place win scored the deciding points to help our girl's team win the CIF 2A Section-Championship trophy.

My coaches and I were happy and grateful because I qualified to jump the following week at the Masters finals meet. This was my amazing achievement after only two years of jumping.

At the CIF Masters meet, I ran the 800 m event and performed the triple-jump. I ran as fast as I could, but I didn't qualify to compete in the State meet. This was a great learning experience to run with the CIF Southern Section's best 800 m runners. I learned how to pace myself like the best, so I could beat them the following year.

At the CIF Masters meet, I also performed the triple-jump. My coaches and I were excited about the results. I finished with the fourth best mark in southern section. I qualified to compete in my first State Championship meet. Unfortunately, I wasn't expected to win one of the six State medals according to the Los Angeles Times Dope Sheet. But I wasn't concerned because I didn't have to run the exhausting 800 m race before I jumped. My body would be energized to execute better than I'd ever done.

At this point of my track career (sophomore year), the State Finals meet was the best athletic experience for me. It was a hot-beautiful day in June. I walked into the huge-packed stadium with nervousness, pride and a big smile because I finally arrived to compete at the "Big Meet" of the year—the coveted State track meet. I was in awe to be one of and amongst the best track and field athletes in California.

Coach Tatum informed me that our sprint relay team needed me, so I ran the second leg of the race. We earned a sixth place medal—my first State medal. I was elated!

After the race, the relay teams received medals. We stood on the sixth place platform, smiled, and waved to the cheering crowds. The official photographer took our pictures. This was an amazing feeling! I thought about returning to the presentation platform for my first state triple-jump medal.

As I walked onto the same blue triple-jump runway, I felt like butterflies were dancing inside my stomach again. I was nervous!

All of the jumpers and I stood in a line (on the runway) and faced the track fans. The crowds were louder than at the recent Masters meet. When the announcer said my name, I looked into the crowded stands, smiled, and waved. Moments later, I saw Coach Taylor in the stands. He smiled and I became emotional with tears in my eyes. I smiled at him with blurry eyes as I thought about all he taught me (in several months) to stand on that state runway— now as a sophomore I was one of the state's best triple-jumpers. I fought back the tears and refocused on executing my six triple-jumps.

Although I was scared, I believed in my mental, running, and jumping abilities. I triple-jumped until the cows came out. I ate, dreamed, and lived with the triple-jump. That day, I believed that I was able to jump farther than 37 feet.

Like the 800 meter run, the competition was fierce. When it ended, I was jumping for joy because I earned another trip to the presentation platform to receive my next State medal. Coach Tatum, Coach Taylor, and I were happy! I placed fifth overall with a personal record of 38 feet 2 inches. That mark surpassed my freshman record by about three feet.

I was one of the happiest athletes at the end of the State Finals! As a sophomore, I went home with two State meet medals and a personal triple-jump record.

Weeks after the state meet, it was time for summer track competitions. Coach Taylor registered me to join a local track club—my initial introduction to age-group track and field competition. It was better than high school track because I competed with athletes in my age group (15-16 year old). He entered my name and marks to compete locally and nationwide.

We traveled to some of the biggest age-group meets in the U.S.A.—San Jose, California, Eugene, Oregon, and St. Louis, Missouri. I won more medals, broke more records, and had more fun. For example, I broke the 800 m record at an age group meet in San Jose. Also, I competed in my first AAU Junior Olympic Games. I won a silver medal in the triple-jump. That experience reminded me of the 1984 Olympic Games in Los Angeles. I planned to return and win the gold medal in the triple jump.

My junior year in high school was amazing! The experience of running and jumping with the best athletes in the prior State meet made me hungrier to return and win. I set goals to win gold medals in the triple jump and 800 meter run in the Pioneer league, CIF finals, and State meets—and break my personal records in each event too.

I worked harder and smarter in practice. I ran faster and with better form. I was stronger and more flexible. I was still running with and scaring the boys in practice. Coach Tatum made me run around the city of Inglewood and took me to the local hills and invitational meets to run. Coach Taylor took me to UCLA and Mt. SAC to jump with talented-male jumpers.

Also, I worked hard in the classroom because my mother expected my sisters and me to get an education. I needed more than a 3.0 G.P.A. for acceptance into college. My mother paid us twenty dollars for A grades and five dollars for B grades. I earned the most of that money. I didn't want to see her for C grades because we'd have a serious meeting that ended with punishment.

Although I was often tired, I completed homework on many bus rides to (and at) basketball games and track meets, and late nights in our small apartment while my family slept. My teammates and coaches knew that education was very important to me. In a 1986 newspaper article, my triple-jump coach said, "She's about a 3.5 (grade point average) in the classroom. She should be a good prospect. If she continues on the pace she's on, she shouldn't have any problems choosing where she wants to go to college."

In the winter season, I was still playing varsity basketball, so I didn't start practice with the track team for indoor or outdoor season (January through June). The last couple track seasons, I started in March. After basketball season, I was glad to be in good shape to fall right into track practice and get into better running and jumping shape.

During basketball season, I was invited to run the 800 m run in one of the coveted indoor meets in America—The Sunkist Invitational Track Meet at the Los Angeles Sports Arena. I was honored to receive the invitation. This meet featured the top-prep runners and jumpers in the state.

This was my first experience running on boards and inside a major sports arena with bright lights and attention. That memorable January evening in the arena, I was the only Morningside High School athlete. It was scary being there without my teammates, but I was glad that Coach Tatum, and my family were there.

I felt like Morningside High School's track star because Wave Newspaper sports editor, Bill Edelstein, interviewed me after my race—my first track interview. He wanted to know how my body felt, who was at the meet with me, how I trained for the meet during a busy-basketball season, and about winning a silver medal at the meet.

While at the arena, I thought about how I overcame flu symptoms that made the prior two weeks of training horrible. But I didn't miss basketball or track practice. My hard work and determination paid off because I won my first indoor-track medal, although I wasn't in track shape.

About a week after the Sunkist track meet, I knew I was officially a local track star. I saw the Edelstein's article with couple paragraphs about me being a forward on my school's (second ranked Division 4A) basketball team and my 800 m race. I was so elated! I made many copies, and shared with my coaches, mother, sisters, best friend, teachers, and everyone who'd listen. They expressed that they were proud of me and to keep up the good work.

About a month later, Edelstein, came to my school to interview me. He asked a lot of questions about my academic, basketball, and track success and goals. He informed me that the article would be published soon.

In February 1987, I ran to find the Wave newspaper in the front yard. When I opened it to the sports section, I saw couple large images of me shooting a basketball and sitting on the bench during a home game. *Althea Moses Morningside's Basketball "Horse" Runs The Fast Track To Success* was the headline below the images. I was overwhelmed with joy because this article was huge. It was about my quick rise and success in academics and athletics.

I had teary eyes when I read, "Althea Moses, track star who has shattered the Morningside 880 record set by Olympian Flo Hyman." Then I broke down with more tears when I read that I owned the Morningside triple-jump record with a leap of 38-5 3/4, and had a 3.7 grade-point average. I wiped my tears away and smiled. I thought about my hard work and dedication to achieve my goals.

I was determined and motivated to reach my academic and athletic goals because the world was watching to see what I'd accomplish next. I wanted to see more of my accomplishments highlighted in more newspapers in order to have the college-track scouts offer me a full-track scholarship.

My junior year-track season was bittersweet. At the league finals, I won gold medals in the 800 m run and triple-jump. I jumped a personal record in the triple-jump (38 ft. 8 1/4 in.). I qualified in both events to return to the CIF prelims.

At the CIF prelims meet, I placed second in the 800 meter run. I won and set the meet record in the triple-jump by more than a foot (39 ft. 9 in.). Both events qualified me to compete in the CIF finals again. I was ecstatic!

On the CIF finals meet day, I walked into stadium with less nervousness as the prior year. I was faster, stronger, and wiser. I was one of the top-prep runners in the California—an official track star.

As I walked onto the track to run the 800 m race, I remembered the last time I almost won a gold 800 m race on it. When the announcer introduced me by name, the crowd cheered louder than the prior year. I was ready and believed I'd win this time, I trained very hard and smart, and I had one of top times in CIF 2A section.

I ran the first curve fast and stayed with the group of runners for the first lap and a half. The race was close like the prior year, but I was fit and determined to win this time. I crossed the finish line first! I felt exhausted. I was happy that tears of joy flooded my eyes as I walked off the track.

When I won, I accomplished one of my 1987 track goals— my running time (2:14.13) was my new personal record. The prior year, I was second in the event. Surprisingly, it was the best 800 m time in the CIF southern section that day—the best qualifying time going into the Masters meet. I felt phenomenal!

What happened next broke my heart. It disturbed my family, coaches, and me because I came into the meet with the best triple jump mark in the CIF Southern Section—also the top three best triple jumper in the country. I was expected to win a gold medal in the event.

Minutes after my 800 m race, I walked over to the triple jump area to complete my run-throughs, but the competition had already commenced. I asked the officials for more time to recover from my race, but it wasn't granted. I didn't consult with Coach Taylor about what to do next. This was a huge mistake and a lesson learned.

I took my first jump and fouled. My foot passed the front of the white board. They showed me how far I was, so I adjusted my run. Then I took my other jumps and fouled. Then my stress level increased because I only had one more jump to win the gold medal and qualify for Masters Meet. I ran down the runway and off the board, hopped, stepped, and long jumped into the sand pit. I felt a sharp pain in my chest as I looked at the red flag waving in the wind. I fouled my final jump.

My heart was broken. I knew that I failed to qualify for a medal and to jump at the Masters meet the following week. This also meant I wouldn't jump in the State meet. My coaches, family, friends, and I were disturbed. I'd learned a valuable lesson—always consult with coaching staff and take time to recover before competing in another event.

My stomach felt sick the rest of the day! I was upset when I read that the best legal triple jump of the day was 37 ft 9 in.—about two feet less than my best (39 ft 9 in.). I had to let that disappointment go and focus on winning the 800 m the next week.

I feel that my CIF triple jump win was sabotaged by certain CIF officials because I came out of nowhere and my triple jump marks surpassed all of the local high school-triple jump marks in a short time. Within couple years, I'd gone from jumping about 33 feet to almost 40 feet without drugs—with great athletic abilities, hard work ethic, determination, and an excellent coaching staff.

The following week at Masters, I ran the 800 m race well. I was excited to have qualified to run at the final meet of the season—1987 CIF State Championships in Sacramento.

At the CIF state meet, I was the only female athlete to compete for my school. I wished my best friend, Ray Wakefield, was there—he always made me laugh. But I wasn't alone because our school's talented boys relay teammates (Eric Frazier, Michael Phillips, Charles Jordan, and Raymond Glass), Coach Tatum, and Coach Estrada were there. We supported each other with respect and kindness. I would've had our coach's full attention, but my teammates earned it too.

Under Coach Tatum and Coach Estrada's training, those boys became some of the top sprinters in California. At the recent CIF 2A Finals, they broke the 400 meter record with 41.11 seconds—had the top time in all divisions in both relays. Also, they won the CIF Division 2A title. At Masters meet final, they upset the state leader (Hawthorne High School) in the event when they beat them in the 400 m relay (41.29) and mile relay (3:13.41). Finally, they had the best mile relay time that night! We were excited!

As a junior, I was elated to return to the State meet to compete for a gold medal in my event. The meet lasted two days. Day one was for qualifying in the top nine marks to compete the next day in the finals. It's also the end of many athlete's season. I was determined not to let my season end on day one.

On the first day, I walked into the huge stadium and felt nervousness. But it didn't last long because I had competed there and won two medals a year ago. I was one of the 800 m track stars to watch.

I stood on my mark on the track. When the starter shot the gun, I ran the curve fast and settled in with the group of runners. I planned to run fast enough to qualify, so I stayed with the runners until the finish line.

After qualifying for day two, I had fun socializing with and watching the other races with few of my track-club friends. I watched the triple-jump event. It was difficult watching the competition that I believed I could've won. But Coach Taylor taught me that I needed to watch to learn how to jump farther. I affirmed to myself, "I'll win it next year."

Day two was the finals championship for medals. I was excited when I walked onto the track to run! The stadium was packed, the crowd was loud, and the weather was hot. I felt that I was ready to execute and win a gold medal.

I stood on my mark confidently. When the gun sounded I ran the first curve fast. I stayed with the group of girls until the last curve. After the first lap and a half, I felt strong and fast, but I didn't increase my speed, because I wanted to be at my strongest and fastest on the last straight to the finish line. But Kim McAllister (top runner from Locke High School) and Hand (Fallbrook) increased their speed on the curve. I maintained my speed and waited to increase it on the last straightaway.

On the straightaway, the race got exciting! I noticed McAllister and Hand started running faster, but not too far ahead of me. The crowd was on their feet and got louder. I ran faster and came closer to Hand. But I couldn't pass McAllister. She crossed the tape first. Hand and I fought hard for second place, but she beat me with a slight lean. That moment was bittersweet for me. I was disappointed with myself for waiting too long to increase my speed and losing the race. I looked up at the timing board and saw that McAllister ran

2:12.92 and Hand 2:13.52. Then I felt excited when I saw my 3rd place time—a new personal record of 2:13.6. I thanked God and my coaches.

Coach Tatum wasn't content with my performance because he believed I was able to win. He congratulated me with a warm smile and hug—then reminded me that I had one more year to win. I believed him.

During the summertime, I remember having fun! Coach Taylor registered me to represent a premiere track club in South Bay. I was the only high school athlete in the club. We traveled with some of El Camino College's top athletes, which included some of Coach Tatum's top performing-former sprinters/hurdlers. I felt right at home.

Couple weeks after the State Meet, we traveled to my first TAC/USA Junior and Intermediate Track and Field Championships (aka Junior Nationals) at University of Arizona. Top prep (Junior) and college athletes competed for national titles and medals in their respective events. It was a pleasure to be in the presence of like-minded and talented young athletes—especially the handsome gentlemen.

We stayed in the college dormitory. This was my first experience staying with college athletes. We had so much fun! I knew that I had to attend college after high school!

Before the triple jump competition commenced, I had the third best mark. I won a silver medal with a mark of 39'10". Then the after-track party commenced!

On the week of 4th of July, I competed in the TAC Youth Nationals at Pennsylvania State University. The weather was hot and humid. I broke my personal 800 m record with a time of 2:13.4 seconds.

Weeks later, I accomplished one of my first major track goals—win an Olympic gold medal. Coach Taylor and I traveled to the AAU Junior Olympic Games at Syracuse University in New York. We stayed in the college dorms with the other athletes and coaches. There were thousands of top-prep athletes in several sports.

At that time, I had experienced that level of competition or athletic event—this event was better. The incredible opening and closing ceremonies blew my mind. It felt like the 1984 Olympics I saw on television. I was pumped up and affirmed that I would win gold and break the Olympic record in the triple jump.

I walked into the huge stadium with wide eyes and much excitement. The crowd was loud. I felt confident. I knew I was healthy, ready to do my best, and have fun. The weather was hot and humid—perfect for jumping far.

During the competition, I had a good series of six jumps. When the final marks were posted, my mark of 40'3/4" placed me in first place. The look on my face said, "Wow!" I was excited that I had just won an Olympic gold medal.

But wait! My excitement escalated when I learned that I'd broken the old Olympic record (39'9 3/4" set in 1981). I jumped up and down with joy and tears. I repeated to myself that I was an Olympic gold medalist and record breaker. I clapped and jumped with joy!

I smiled at Coach Taylor as he stood in the stands. He was pacing and smiling with excitement too. I could see that he was proud of me—his first Olympic gold medalist and record breaker. Moments like that were what we dreamed, planned, and worked hard to make reality. Let's not forget making sacrifices for, too.

The other girl jumpers were happy for me too. They congratulated me with kind words and hugs. Some wanted to know about my training routine. I felt that Coach Taylor and I should start a triple-jump clinic.

That Olympic victory gave me one of the best feelings I'd experienced. I'll never forget it. That win was redemption for me—after failing to qualify at CIF Finals Meet two months prior. I thanked God Almighty for redemption.

Upon my return home, the City of Inglewood (The City of Champions) recognized my Olympic achievements with splendor. Mayor Edward Vincent, Jr. and the City Council honored several community members and me at the 4th Annual Community Unity Awards Dinner. It was awesome! I enjoyed the event with my family and Coach Taylor. As someone read my biography aloud, my eyes filled with tears and my heart and mouth smiled. Then, they awarded me with an official City of Inglewood certificate in a large-gold frame. It looks great on my office wall.

My senior year in high school was absolutely amazing! I was one of the top prep athletes in the country—an Olympic gold medalist and record breaker in the triple jump. But I wasn't a state champion yet. I wanted to be a State champion, so I set goals and worked very hard. I often affirmed, "I will win more gold medals and break more records in the triple jump and 800 meter run in league, CIF finals, and State meet."

In the fall of 1987 (before basketball and track season), I ran cross-country for the first time. I disliked training and running three miles nonstop, but I believed that it'd strengthen my endurance for the 800 m run. Surprisingly, I won a silver medal in league finals and qualified for the CIF prelims. The following week, I ran well, but didn't qualify to run in the CIF finals for cross-country. My cross-country season ended.

After cross-country season, I returned to train for my final year as a forward on our award-winning-varsity basketball team. Lisa Leslie was our center.

That final year in high school (1987), I didn't enjoy playing on our team because I felt unneeded. The team had four other talented starting girls and back up on the bench, so I told Coach Scott that I'm leaving the team. He appeared to be surprised. After all, I'd played on his team since my freshman year.

I returned my team uniforms and bag and informed Coach Scott that I plan to focus my time and energy on track and field because I want to win gold medals in the State meet. He accepted my decision, but didn't stop there. I felt that he needed me to win the state basketball championship, so he spoke to my track coaches. Fortunately, I respected my coaches and believed that I could help the basketball team and win my gold medals in the State track meet too.

In 1987, my schedule was very busy! After basketball and track practices and on weekends, I worked at Wendy's Hamburger Restaurant, completed homework and research projects, and studied for exams. My social life was minimal. Ray was a hurdler on our team, so we spent time at his family's home, while talking about track and field, and listening to music by the legend, Prince.

Why did I work? I like the best of things, but my mother couldn't afford to purchase the gold jewelry, Gucci and Louis Vuitton bags, Guess jeans, and Nike tennis shoes that I desired. She suggested that I get a job, so I did. When I got paid, my mother didn't expect me to help with her bills. I often donated some of my income to her and my grandmother.

In the end of 1987, I was invited to run the invitational 800 m run in the coveted 1988 Sunkist Indoor Invitational Meet again. This thrilled me because it was an opportunity to beat Kim McAllister—1987 State Meet 800 m champion. So, I was on a mission to listen and do whatever Coach Tatum told me to run.

After basketball practice ended (nighttime), Coach Tatum took me to train on the dirt track at Fox Hills Park. It was about the same distance as the 800 m run. I was determined and often affirmed that I would beat McAllister at the L.A. Sports Arena.

Training for the 800 m race wasn't easy because I was always tired after attending six classes and practicing couple hours in the gym. Additionally, the winter nights were so cold and Coach Tatum's workout regimen was tough! I worked very hard! For instance, I had to run certain times for every race, or I'd hear the firm, "Come on Moses!"

After my nighttime practice, Coach Tatum drove me to our apartment in the Bottoms (urban area in Inglewood). I ate dinner, completed homework, showered, and went to sleep. Then repeat all of it the next day. I often affirmed, "I'll beat Kim!"

I was nervous and excited as I stood on the escalator to the basement floor of the Los Angeles Sports Arena. I warmed up well. I was ready to run my best 800 m race. Coach Tatum reminded me about my strategy and goal to win.

The starter's gun sounded and most of the runners and I ran quickly to set the pace. I remained close to Kim and the other girls. They increased their speed and I did the same.

On the final lap of our race, Kim increased her speed like she did in the State meet. However, this race was different because I increased my speed too. I wasn't ready to sprint ahead of her. I ran on her right side. She appeared to be concerned, so she started pushing me away with her right arm. I was surprised with her behavior. However, I didn't push back. I kept running next to her with my left arm in front of me—to avoid touching her.

The crowd was on their feet and cheering loudly. We continued running side by side. As we ran on the back straight and toward the final curve, I increased my speed. About a second later, Kim fell off the track. I didn't stop or look back. I continued running by myself to the finish line. I looked over to see how Kim was doing.

I was excited that I'd beaten the State champ as planned. Minutes later, my excitement turned to heartbreak. A meet official held up a red flag and disqualified me from my gold medal performance. He said that I pushed Kim during the race. No, that's untrue! I watched video footage of that race. It's clear that she was pushing me and I ran with my left arm in front of me. I believe that as Kim kept pushing me from the inside lane, she placed her left foot off the track and slipped. Furthermore, I wasn't a person who harmed others for my personal gain. After all, my mother raised me to be honest, work hard, and treat others the way I want to be treated.

My family, friends, and coaches congratulated me. They said (from their position in the stands) they saw Kim pushing me, I was avoiding her, and she felt off the track.

During the track season, I felt like a track star because some sports writers came to my school and track meets to interview me. I recall feeling like a star whenever I was featured (with action pictures) in the sports section of the Wave Newspaper and Los Angeles Times Newspaper.

After the Sunkist Meet, I continued training and playing with our talented basketball team. Throughout the season, we were undefeated in league. We won our league finals and CIF League Championship. As a result of the CIF win, we qualified to play in the coveted CIF regional finals at the Sports Arena. Ironically, that final local game positioned me to return to the Los Angeles Sports Arena floors—where I beat Kim McCallister several months prior. This experience was bittersweet because I was happy to play with my team at the Sports Arena and had to wait another couple weeks before starting my training with the track team.

The following week, we beat Lynwood High School at the Los Angeles Sports Arena. It was a sweet victory because they were as talented as we were. After the game ended, we celebrated on the court like the NBA players do at the finals. This win qualified us for the coveted CIF State Championship Finals game in Oakland, California.

Our team arrived at the Oakland Sports Arena with excitement. I was excited and nervous. We played against a talented group of girls from an Oakland high school. We worked hard to beat them.

The final few minutes of the game got really intense! We needed to score the last basket to win the championship. I was exhausted because I played most of the game. Oakland wasn't giving up. They were playing like the boys and men at the outdoor parks. Unfortunately, we lost the championship game by one point. In that final game, I didn't feel good about how I was treated by some of my teammates. I was glad that basketball season ended. Immediately, I started thinking about the work I needed to do to earn a full track scholarship to UCLA, break meet records, and win gold medals at CIF Finals and the California Track and Field Championships in June.

The week after returning from Oakland, I was ready to transition to track practice. Being in good shape from basketball season made a huge difference in practice.

I trained harder and smarter, and ran faster with better form. I ran and jumped with the boys in practice. Some of the boys were still scared of me running past, or jumping farther than them.

After track practice, I worked harder in the weight room. It made me stronger. Often, I performed plyometrics (jump training). It made me more explosive off the ground. Also, I made better effort to consume healthier foods and drink more water.

League finals came faster than the prior years. I had fun winning gold medals in the triple jump and 800 m run—they qualified me to defend my gold-medal titles in the CIF finals.

At the CIF Finals meet, I had fun defending my 800 m run medal. I won a gold medal. After the race, I didn't make the mistake made the prior year. I took more time to recover before competing in the triple jump event. I warmed up well and focused on executing like the champion I was.

After six jumps, I won the gold in the triple jump. It was sweet redemption after failing to qualify the prior year. My tears flowed onto my cheeks as I placed my track spikes into my bag. I smiled and waved proudly at the crowd as I stood on the first place platform and received my gold medal. As a result, I qualified for the Masters Final in the 800 m run and triple jump.

The following week at the Masters meet finals, I won the triple jump and qualified for the coveted State meet finals. I cried tears of joy on the track. I was set to jump in the State Championships the next weekend!

After the meet, I rushed home and got dressed to attend the senior prom. I arrived about an hour before it ended, so I was only able to take pictures with my prom date. Then I got dressed to enjoy the after-prom event.

The week before the State finals, disagreements occurred between couple of my track coaches. Coach Taylor was training and competing in the triple jump to qualify for the 1988 Olympics. He had a scheduling conflict. Taylor couldn't attend our State championship meet because he was scheduled to compete in Europe. When he informed me, I felt scared, but understood because he was pursuing his dream of being an Olympian while he trained his athletes.

The news of Taylor leaving didn't go well at Morningside High School. Coach Taylor said Coach Estrada expressed to him that he should be at the meet with me. He informed him that it was unnecessary because he believed in my keen focus and abilities, and that I was prepared to win without him. Taylor said that I understood that track had to come first. I could prioritize everything to execute and become a champion.

I understood Coach Estrada's point, but agreed with Coach Taylor. I was confident that I was ready and able to execute and win at the State meet. After all, I was focused, determined to win, and had jumped forty-plus feet in practice and other meets.

At the State track and field finals (Cerritos College), the stadium was packed and the fans were cheering. I smiled as I walked onto the blue runway with confidence. I saw some girls staring at me with fright in their eyes. They watched me measure my runway mark from the thirty-six foot board, perform run throughs, and no step approaches into the sandbox.

Some girls came to congratulate me on my recent CIF and Masters meet wins. Others said they were amazed with my triple-jump form. Some asked how I was able to jump from a thirty-six feet board because most girls jumped from the thirty and thirty-two feet boards. I smiled and responded, "I practiced until the cows came out."

I believed that I could win the triple jump because I won league, CIF, and Masters Meet finals. I was healthy and focused on executing my six jumps well.

After six jumps, I won the gold medal with almost forty-one feet (40' 9 ¾"). I became Morningside's first State (Triple Jump) gold-medal champion, and extended my school record in the triple jump. My tears rolled down my cheeks, and I was overcome with immense joy and gratitude! I thanked God, my mother, and all three coaches for helping me earn a CIF State Track and Field gold medal!

In June, I graduated with cum laude honors with 3.6 cumulative G.P.A—number six in my graduating class. I was elated and proud about earning a UCLA track and field scholarship. My mother was proud of me too. I felt great because my hard work paid off and some of my dreams were accomplished.

MY COLLEGE EXPERIENCE

The second year of college my personal life and health was impacted harshly. I had a boyfriend who physically abused me. One day we had a disagreement. He grabbed my jacket, lifted me off the street, and slammed me against his car. The impact was powerful, I felt excruciating pain in my back, neck, and head. I got flashbacks of daddy physically abusing my mother. I fought back. He released me as he called me a bitch. I immediately broke up with him.

Weeks later, this now ex-boyfriend broke into my apartment when I was away. As I spoke to the police about the incident, he walked up and admitted to breaking in. They arrested him and took him to jail. I got a restraining order to keep him away from me. I moved on with my life, but feared him for many years.

My student-athlete years at UCLA were bittersweet. My first couple years were frustrating because the triple jump workouts didn't include bounding on the grass, over hurdles or boxes. It was mostly springboard workouts into the sandbox. As a result, I could barely jump forty feet, like in high school.

I informed the head and jump coaches that I needed to bound in order to jump forty plus feet. The head coach, Bob Kersee, told me to follow their program. I did. During my freshman and sophomore year, I failed to surpass my personal record (40'9 3/4") in the triple jump. I was frustrated, so I focused on graduating with a UCLA degree. For fun, I socialized with my buddy—track star, Janeene.

At my first PAC-10 Finals, I struggled to jump more than 40'9 3/4". I felt bad because some of the girls that I beat in high school were jumping forty-plus feet. Before departing from the track, I cried with frustration! My heart was broken and I longed to jump farther, like a champion again. After the event, Kersee apologized to me. I felt it was due to not allowing me to bound as I requested.

The next year, Kersee's action made me very happy. He hired Coach Yendork to train the jumpers. Yendork's training was similar to my former triple jump coach in high school. He trained his daughter (State triple-jump champion) and many other jumpers to surpass the forty feet mark. His workouts were fun and grueling—they included bounding on the grass and runway, over/onto hurdles, and boxes. He also instructed his athletes to execute no-step to six-step approach triple jumping and sprinting after those grueling workouts. Then we lifted weights and did more plyometric exercises in the weight room (Bruin Brawn).

In 1993 and 1995, Belize chose me to triple jump in the World Championship in Athletics. It's an honor I cherish! I traveled to Stuttgart, Germany and Gothenburg, Sweden. I resided in the Athlete's Village with the world's best track and field athletes. I met, dined, and partied with many of whom I read about or saw on television. The experience was amazing in many ways. Often, the locals stopped me for my autograph and to take pictures with them. I felt like a star!

At both World Championship meets, I jumped forty-plus feet, but didn't win any medals. The experience was unforgettable because I competed with the world's best triple-jumpers. I'm ecstatic that my name and marks are in the World Championship archives forever.

As a senior at UCLA, I had another boyfriend who physically abused me. I told him I was moving on, so he slapped me hard--I saw stars! Then he punched me in my right ribcage. I grabbed my stomach and hunched over in pain. He apologized. I didn't tell anyone. I was unable to practice due to pain I experienced. Note: To this day, I have scar tissue in that area.

My final years (1992 and 1993) at UCLA were sweet because I started jumping more than forty-one feet. I won a silver trophy at the PAC-10 Finals meet. Also, I broke my personal record with more than forty-one feet! My marks placed me on the UCLA Top-Ten-Triple-Jumper List.

After my senior year at UCLA, I was invited to jump as a professional athlete at the 1996 Modesto Invitational Meet. I placed second and earned a $500 check. That year, my personal best triple-jump mark was 12.79 meters (42'8 3/4").

Coach Yendork informed me that he was leaving UCLA for another position, so I became frightened. This was the start of my thirteenth year of training for the Olympics, so I prayed to God that he'd guide me to a good coach to continue jumping forty-two feet plus—mark needed to qualify for the Olympic Games.

Not long after, I hired Greg Harper to train me. I trusted him. He was a kind and an accomplished USC triple-jumper. We trained hard at USC. It was fun in practice because of the UCLA vs USC rivalry. I jumped about 42 feet.

THE OLYMPIC GAMES EXPERIENCE

In 1996, I was elated that my dreams of becoming a three-time Olympian and jumping on the world's biggest athletic stage had become reality. I received the call from the Belize Olympic Committee. I was one of five athletes who qualified to compete in the 1996 Centennial Summer Olympic Games. It's known officially as the Games of the XXVI Olympiad.

This major international multi-sport event took place in Atlanta, Georgia (USA). I lived and trained in Los Angeles, so I traveled to Atlanta via plane. I met the Belize Olympic delegation at the huge Olympic Village. It was on a university campus in Atlanta. This was the venue where most of the athletes and their delegations resided, dined, socialized, and practiced for the Games. It wasn't too far away from the AT&T Village—downtown where the bombing occurred during the Games.

I enjoyed life at the Village because I love to eat good food! The kitchen was huge and amazing because it served foods from all over the world—it was open twenty-four hours a day. To my delight, there was a McDonald's Restaurant serving free food and drinks twenty-hour hours. After my event ended, I ate so many delicious Big Macs, chicken nuggets, fries, and soft serve cones. After thirteen years of sacrifice, hard work, and diet restrictions, I was excited to treat my mouth well.

The Olympic opening ceremony was held at the Centennial Olympic Stadium in Atlanta, GA (now Turner Field). It was unforgettable. For more than couple hours, each country's delegation walked and waited in long lines outside of the Olympic stadium.

At first, it was exciting to wait until I started sweating profusely in my uniform. All of the Belizean athletes were given a navy-polyester coat with our Belize Olympic logo on the front. We looked great as a team. However, the torrid weather made me feel uncomfortable. While we waited, we took pictures, exchanged our country's Olympic pins, and socialized with other Olympians.

When we entered the huge, Olympic stadium, the fans cheered loudly. I could barely hear my teammates call my name. I was ecstatic when I heard the announcer introduce the Belize delegation. I cried with immense joy as I walked and waved at the fans. Through the tears, I saw other athletes with tears in their eyes. When some of our eyes connected, we smiled and gave each other the thumbs up—gesturing congratulations and you did it!

After the final delegation arrived into the stadium, the crowd cheered louder. I love this historic experience!

One of the most memorable Olympic moments occurred during the opening ceremony. Speculation grew leading up to the ceremony about who'd light the Olympic flame in the cauldron. The identity of the person to light it was kept a secret, so I waited anxiously.

On the track, I saw Olympic gold medalist Janet Evans and Evander Holyfield holding an Olympic torch. They jogged toward a girl waiting for them to light her torch. They lit her torch. Then she jogged onto a platform to light the torch of the 1960 Olympic gold medalist and former American-professional boxer and activist, Muhammad Ali.

I was in awe to see Ali in person for the first time. Along with the audience, I cheered and clapped loudly! Ali raised his torch to the fans. The audience clapped and yelled, "Ali! Ali! Ali!" The crowds cheered and clapped louder. He turned and lit the Olympic cauldron. It was a memorable moment showing Ali's will despite having Parkinson's disease.

Another memorable Olympic moment was having my mother supporting me at the stadium and in the Olympic Village. Initially, my mother was unable to travel to see me compete in the Olympics due to lack of money for a plane ticket. However, her coworkers decided that she should be there. They donated money for her to purchase a plane ticket to see me compete in the Olympic Games. I enjoyed spending time with her. We took a lot of pictures and dined in the huge Olympic kitchen. Also, I'm grateful that she was there to see me jump in my final track meet.

As I entered the stadium to compete, I recalled (as a freshman in high school) telling many people that I was going to the Olympics—although the triple jump wasn't a medaled Olympic event for women. I believed that it'd become an Olympic event for us because girls and women were jumping farther than previous years. Then it became reality in 1996—I was competing there. I smiled and said, "Wow!"

The day came when my name was called to line up with the other triple-jumpers to compete on the Olympic stage. As I walked in our line, my excited spirit trembled and my tears of joy welled up in my eyes. I looked up and took in a 360 view of the huge stadium with thousands of fans. Their cheers were loud. I felt amazing and accomplished.

It was amazing to be there! I felt nervous for a short time. Then I felt confident and proud to be on that Olympic runway to do what I enjoyed doing—triple-jumping and entertaining the global track and field fans.

After executing my three jumps, I finished with high forty-one feet marks. However, it wasn't sufficient to win one of the three medals. However, I didn't cry about it. I was happy because I lived my dream of triple jumping in the 1996 Summer Olympics. I'm grateful that Belize and Althea Gilharry Moses names and marks are in the Olympic archives forever.

There's one unmemorable moment that shakes my spirit when recalled—the deadly terrorist attack on <u>Centennial Olympic Park</u> in Atlanta. I spent several hours having lots of fun at this location. I felt sleepy, so I rode a shuttle back to the Olympic Village and fell asleep.

The next morning, I learned of the deadly attack while watching the news. My tears welled up in my eyes, and my spirit trembled as I thought about the victims, and how God removed me from the AT&T Village about an hour before the explosion occurred there. I thank God when I remember it.

After the Olympics, I returned to my apartment in Inglewood. My mother rewarded me with a memorable t-shirt that had a picture of me triple jumping in Europe. She had it made to thank her coworkers—and suggested wearing it while viewing the Olympic opening ceremony and my competition on television. Thanks, Concepts former staff!

I accepted that my thirteen-years of determination, hard work, and sacrifice to live my Olympic dream were done. I hoped that the five Belize Olympians would've received an acknowledgment from the Belizean community in Belize and Los Angeles. I haven't received the Prime Minister of Belize's invitation to visit the government house. The Belize Olympic Committee and Belize consulate haven't acknowledged my Olympic achievement with an award, or organized event celebration. I'm still the Belize national record holder in the triple-jump and other events.

Since the Olympics, I've earned a Masters degree in Education and California Professional Clear Teaching Credential. I've established businesses in real estate, health and fitness, and consultation.

As I prepared to publish this book, I asked Coach Estrada about my motivation when he trained me. He said I didn't need motivation. I was motivated by my desire to succeed and leave the tough-urban neighborhood—sometimes with teenaged pregnancies, gangs, gang-related deaths, and noisy emergency sirens and planes. He was impressed by my positive response and determination to pursue my dreams of being successful in the midst of distractions.

Estrada reminded me of my senior year routine as a poor-teenage dreamer. In the fall, winter, and spring, my daily routine included walking to all of the following places: school for grueling morning-cross country practice, six classes, and grueling basketball and track practices. Then I walked to Wendy's Hamburger Restaurant, where I worked several hours. At the end of many nights, I was mentally and physically exhausted!

I believed and decided that quitting wasn't an option—and education was the key to leave "the hood" or neighborhood. My mother was very supportive and didn't play with my four sisters and me! She expected her daughters to get an education and A and B grades in order to graduate from high school. Since she paid us cash for good grades, I didn't sleep until my homework and studying were completed.

Estrada expressed that anyone with that much determination doesn't need to be motivated. They just need someone in their corner. He said that individuals like me motivated him.

Coach Tatum expressed, "MHS students and coaches were dedicated and committed to working to be CIF and State champions." I'm glad I was apart of that incredible-unforgettable legacy.

Collectively with my three former high school coaches' track and field knowledge, dedication, and support, my tenacity, commitment, hard work, and drive to win, and my mother's love and support, I became a true champion.

I'm so glad that I was blessed to start my track career with the knowledge, love, dedication, and support of my former three coaches—Ronald Tatum, Johnny Estrada, Darryl Taylor. They, along with my mother, inspired me to be a champion in academics and athletics. She taught me to get an education and to believe I can do whatever I put my mind to and to never give up. Getting an education became our household anthem.

My high-school track coaches laid my strong, rock- solid bodybuilding foundation. They taught me how to build my teenage body through running and jumping exercises on the track, beach, hills, pool, and weight-training exercises. They expected all track athletes to walk straight to the weight room after track workouts.

Coach Tatum, Taylor, and Estrada showed they cared about our success by not allowing us to do what we wanted. They expected us to listen, follow directions, perform required running workout times, and always show up—do whatever it took (legally) to become champions and productive citizens in the world. If we didn't show up to the track or weight room, someone was sent to find us, and consequences provided if disappearing became a habit.

I got extensive knowledge and practice about weight training and its benefits. For example, I learned weight-training terms: sets, repetitions, pyramid, routine. I learned how to use barbells, dumbbells, and cabled machines. I learned the exercise techniques needed to safely perform these strength/weight training exercises: squat, lunges, leg extensions, leg curls, toe raises, shoulder raises, triceps extensions, bench press, arm curls, dips between benches, sit ups, crunches, leg raises, and more. You'll perform many of these exercises in your routine.

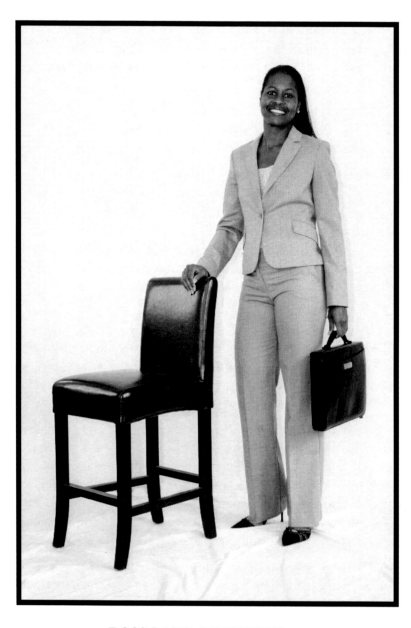

BOSS LADY OF FITNESS ™

"For we are the temple of the living God."
(2 Corinthians 6:16 NIV Bible)

CHAPTER 2

HOW TO BUILD AND STRENGTHEN YOUR SPIRIT

Many people fail to be aware that their spirit needs exercising to be healthy too. This chapter will bring awareness and methods to help you become spiritually strong, or stronger than before.

On my eighteen-year-spiritual journey, I've been building and strengthening my spirit, daily, with ancient, modern, and/or traditional and non-traditional spiritual approaches—believing, studying, embracing, and practicing incredible mind and spiritual exercises. More people are integrating both processes and/or approaches into their lives. Studies show that practicing both approaches are working well for many people. For more than a decade, it's been working for my clients and me. Before sharing all of my spiritual exercises, I'll share my incredible spiritual journey with you to be inspired.

One of the first important aspects of spiritual strengthening I've embraced is inner light. In my adulthood with all its joys and sufferings, I learned and believe that God's light dwells within me. I'm not alone with this belief. Many wise people have expressed it too. "Use the light that dwells within you to regain your natural clarity of sight," said Lao Tzu, Chinese philosopher.

Dr. Michael Bernard Beckwith, author of *Spiritual Liberation: Fulfilling Your Soul's Potential,* said, "And yet few of us even know that this inner light exists let alone that we may access and apply it to our spiritual, mental, emotional, creative, or physical life structures." That's one of the things I've done on my journey—used my light to strengthen and maintain my mind, spirit, and body temple, and inspire others to do the same.

Every day, people all over the world awaken to their personal health and spiritual practices or exercises, along their life journey. Quite often, most are unconscious about it, and don't consider the health or wellbeing of the internal part of their body, mind, and spirit.

I've successfully strengthened my mind and spirit. I recommend building your mind and spirit by incorporating daily mind and spiritual exercises before eating breakfast, leaving your home, or building your body temple. Those spiritual exercises will set the tone for the rest of your day. You'll become stronger, happier, more energized, focused, and fulfilled.

After all, you know your body temple will die. But what will become of your inner spirit? I believe it'll live eternally. While your spirit is within your body temple, let's make it strong or stronger with traditional and nontraditional exercises to enjoy all of the benefits they offer.

I've experienced positive results from yoga exercises, fasting, chanting, meditating, and praying to cleanse and strengthen my spirit. I was elated to learn that many ancient traditions consider internal cleansing and strengthening of the mind, body, and spirit. They help to achieve total clarity and empowerment of the body.

The following ancient healing and health practices offer the following: the practice of yoga executes cleansing practices called *shuddhi kriyas* to assist in total purification of the body. Christianity engages in fasting and praying to God and Jesus. Buddhism performs chanting. Islam engages in fasting and Ramadan. Judaism engages in *Mikvah.* "The *mikvah* is a body of water where a person immerses themselves and starts to meditate and have certain thoughts and ideas. He uses these ideas, while he's submerging himself in the water, to realize his potential for actualization," explains Yonah Akiva, a lifelong Judaism student on KITV News.

At about age thirty, I was fed up with how some of my love ones mistreated and defined me. I began attending church to learn what the Bible said about intimate relationships and me. I learned a lot at Faithful Central Bible Church in Inglewood. Bishop Ulmer's Bible sermons prompted me to do my own research to discern what the Bible said about who I am, what my purpose was, and how I could make a difference, or change the world for the better.

The few years as a member at Faithful Central were bittersweet, but transformational. It was a springboard to learning more about spirituality, relationships, and myself—how what people believe and practice impact their beliefs, behaviors, and lives.

Importantly, I left the church knowing who I am, and my spirit began to get strong.

Since then, I learned about other religions and spiritual practices, which transformed the way I think about religion, others, and myself. I believe that focusing on self-improvement and spirituality with daily spiritual practices has made a significant difference in my life. I call them "exercises" because they help to strengthen and maintain my spirit, like physical exercises do for my firm-body temple. With consistency, they'll do the same for you.

On your journey, I recommend disallowing people from defining who you are. During the initial part of my spiritual journey, some people defined who I was based on my achievements, place of birth, faith, and physical appearance. That didn't strengthen my spirit, or enhance my happiness.

At age thirty, I defined myself for myself. Who am I? I'm a child of God—not a Christian or religious. Defining yourself for yourself will strengthen your spirit, and empower you to deal with people who may define who you are. Also, it'll prevent people from informing you to do the following: what style and color of clothes, shoes, and makeup to wear, how often to attend the church building, how much money to give to the church, what type of person to date or marry.

I've learned to use mantra, meditation, and prayers to achieve and maintain a strong spirit. It has been rock solid for almost two decades. Although I believe in the Creator God and prayed regularly, I was unsure if I was practicing mantra and meditation. My research helped to enlighten me. I was practicing mantra, but not meditation. I started meditations, and my spirit felt stronger.

For your spiritual strengthening, I recommend the daily usage of *mantra*—every morning for about a minute. M*antra* is a basic method that guides you to your source of thought like a rocket. I meditate at six AM. According to a report, Oprah Winfrey (former host of *The Oprah Winfrey Show* and chairwoman, CEO, and CCO of the *Oprah Winfrey Network*) and her staff meditate at nine AM and five PM. The staff at Agape International Spiritual Center in California has weekday meditation at three PM, according to

Akili Beckwith (manager of *Alice's Quiet Mind Bookstore* at Agape).

I recommend the daily usage of *meditation*. *Meditation* is a basic mental technique that stills your mind and body. It allows you and the Creator God to communicate with each other. Every religion uses *meditation*. It doesn't matter what you believe, you can meditate—sit still, close your eyes, breathe normal, and quietly communicate with God, or your inner child. Ask God about His intentions for you.

I recommend the daily usage of *prayer*. *Prayer* is the basic method of talking and singing to and/or with the Creator God— aloud or quietly.

Prayers have strengthened my mind and spirit, and work to help me feel better through the good and troubling times of my life. However, in 2011-2012, my prayers weren't working fast enough when I was blindsided by betrayal of my trust. I learned that my then-fiancé was involved in a relationship with a former girlfriend.

All of a sudden, I felt unbalanced. My body was firm, but my spirit felt weak. The anguish of betrayal didn't feel well for a while. I needed something else to push past self-doubt, fear of losing him, weakness, and temptations.

A friend advised me to consider the addition of the Ho'oponopono practice for faster relief. I did extensive research. Ho'oponopono is an ancient Hawaiian practice of reconciliation and forgiveness. It has self-healing exercises, or practices of self-identity. It includes prayers, meditation, and four fundamental ideas or phrases. I felt comfortable with the idea of praying and saying the phrases, but meditation was challenging.

I decided to practice the Ho'oponopono exercises. I believed they'd help to strengthen my spirit and overcome my anguish. On the first day of practice, I felt peaceful, cleansed, and rebalanced. I was amazed about how strong I felt on the first day of practicing the exercises! Since then, I practice them daily.

Practicing Ho'oponopono enlightened me. It taught me to love, forgive, apologize, and be thankful in spite of what I perceived as bad or negative memories. I learned to be free from all bad memories, data, and information, and love unconditionally. I recommend practicing Ho'oponopono too.

NOTE: Ho'oponopono practice and my personal story of overcoming troubling times are in one of my next books.

Indeed, my exercising (mind and spirit) occurs during Quiet Time—a time to be with the Creator. Sometimes it occurs in the afternoon, or evenings. I pray, meditate, say my mantra, and read and study scriptures in my Bible. I say my declarations and affirmations, and Ho'oponopono prayers, meditations, and cleansing list. I've memorized all of them due to several years of daily practice.

Exercising my spirit with those very important exercises sets the tone for the rest of my day. My spirit is rock-solid. No matter what happens to my body temple, everything is all right with my spirit. I possess mindfulness through those practices. I'm fulfilled. Whenever I didn't show up to Quiet Time, I felt the opposite experience—unhappy, unfocused, and unfulfilled.

You should make every effort to keep your spirit strengthening commitment to yourself as you would with any personal or business appointment on your calendar. Indeed, maintaining your strong spirit and body temple is important because you want them to remain rock solid. I look at it like a job, or intimate relationship that's important to me. I'll do whatever I think and/or feel is necessary not to lose them.

Daily communication with the Divine makes all the difference in the world to me, and it will for you too. Have an opened mind, spirit, and heart. It helps to quiet or calm your spirit—which promotes internal health and wellbeing.

In order to experience sustaining results, you need to believe in the higher power. That something that's bigger than you and everything—the one sure source and resource of your life. I call him God, Creator, Abba. It's worth believing in a higher power. HD Watson, poet, stated to me that the longest travel in life is the journey within oneself. I agree. Start practicing the exercises in this book to strengthen your spirit today. Enjoy them and the journey within yourself—to your happiest.

Another exercise that strengthens my spirit is practicing gratitude daily. I feel that it's the greatest emotion to have. In spite of experiencing my spirit and body temple shaken, I'm grateful. Thank God for everything you have, and the good and negative thoughts, perceptions, beliefs, and memories.

As a result of possessing a strong spirit, I've experienced amazing conscious results that have caused me to feel better about myself and make better choices in all aspects of my life. For example, saying no and being authentic with others without fear of losing them.

I believe that God created each of us for His good purpose. I feel my purpose is to help people (globally) who are willing to work to improve their lives, through spirituality, health, wellness, fitness, and business ownership. This is my treasure and passion and where my heart is daily. It makes me happy and free whenever I think about, and am doing it too. It's written, "For where your treasure is, there your heart will be also." (Matthew 6:21 NIV Bible)

Since you desire to build and strengthen your spirit, you should practice as many of the mind, body, and spirit exercises in this book. Ask the Creator God what's His intention for your life—and to guide you into all understanding and equip you to do good works. It's written, "All scripture is God-breathed and useful for teaching, rebuking, correcting, and training in righteousness, so that the man of God may be thoroughly equipped for every good work. (2 Timothy 3:16-17 NIV)

Make a commitment to your daily spiritual exercising. It will strengthen your mind and spirit when you consistently apply it. A commitment to your spiritual practice can enlighten your life and help you forgive easier.

Here's an essential tip: after praying or communicating with the Divine God and saying your affirmations and declarations, breathe deeply. Hold it around your expanded awareness, positive thoughts, and intentions. Release it when you're ready. It calibrates your nervous system and conscious mind to accept what you stated, according to Dr. Michael Bernard Beckwith. It works. I feel so free when and after communicating with the Creator God—almost two decades now.

For the past several years, I've experienced many manifestations of what I affirmed and declared daily. For example, completion of this book, my book becoming a bestseller, producing and hosting a live radio show, speaking at big events, teaching my trademarked mind, body, and spirit exercise (*ALTHEA*), and being an inspiration to all audiences.

According to, Diana Vela, people should lead with their spiritual life, highest being, highest consciousness, and heart. They should also bring to life the full expression of their being first, and always.

"Lead with your spiritual life. Something has to be first," said Rod McIver. What a nice quote.

I lead with my heart and my spiritual life. I'm happy and free to be me. The Creator God's guiding and blessing me on my journey. Remember that your spirit requires work as does your body temple—and not only on Sundays. Step forward and start exercising now.

Here are some examples of my Quiet Time, or spirit strengthening exercises—prayers, mantra, and meditations. Every morning, I choose several of the exercises before leaving my home. I recommend that you exercise with these to become spiritually strong too.

I sit on the edge of my bed with my feet off the floor. I say, "I love you, Divine God, Abba, Jesus, Holy Spirit, angels, Inner Child (Little Althea), Divine Heart, and ancestors. Then I stand up and say **The Lord's Prayer**, like a child talking to their parents. I'm informing the Creator God of my appreciation and gratitude for all of my gifts or blessings—which includes my strong spirit and firm-body temple.

The Lord's Prayer

Our Father in heaven,

Hallowed be your name,

your kingdom come,

your will be done,

on earth as it is in heaven.

Give us today our daily bread.

And forgive us our debts,

as we also have forgiven our debtors.

And lead us not into temptation,

but deliver us from the evil one.

(Matthew 6: 9-13 NIV)

Then I pray with these words and more. "God, thank you for your sweet rest, waking me again, protection, renewal of my mind, salvation, and all you've done for my family and me."

Next, I pray one to three personally created prayers:

Prayer #1

God, please continue to remove the darkness that has been covering my family, friends, and me. Make it disappear forevermore. Make your light shine upon us forevermore. Show the people around us how you bless the righteous. Help us to resist as you destroy all the evil desires of our enemies. Bring us a great end to this year. Fulfill all of our needs and help us overcome all of our trials, forevermore. And it is done. Amen.

Prayer #2 (Inspired by the Jabez Prayer in the Bible)

Oh that you would bless my family, friends, and me indeed. Please enlarge our territories and the territories of all active business owners to prosperous networks. Please keep your right hand with us and protect your children, places, and things in the world, from harm, evil, and injury that there's no pain caused by or to us. And it is done. Amen.

Prayer #3

God, please bless me with excellent retention of all that I read, hear, and see—with wisdom, knowledge, understanding, and a discerning heart that I may do your will, let your goodness shine, lead, help, and teach your people, forevermore. And it is done. Amen.

MY MANTRA

I am what I am.

I am God's child.

I'm happy, healthy, wealthy, powerful, strong, protected, cherished, and loved.

I am what I am.

MY PERSONAL DECLARATIONS

I, Althea Moses, declare:

I am dearly loved and cherished forever.

I can do no wrong.

I have nothing to fear.

My heart is opened to the wonders of love and life.

I love, cherish, and honor myself as the precious soul I am.

I live a very prosperous, happy, healthy, wealthy, safe, generous, and loving life.

MY PERSONAL AFFIRMATION

I am involved in God consciousness.

God show me what to deliver today.

Clear my mind to hear you today.

Life is for me. Life is you.

Everything works together for my good and your glory.

I have freedom, joy, peace, and God.

My problems are helping me to birth who I am:

A dearly loved and cherished, happy, protected, and grateful child of God.

I am strong, brave, courageous, and fearless.

The grace of our Lord Jesus and God is with me.

I have everything I want.

And it's done.

HO'OPONOPONO SPIRITUAL PRACTICE

(Inspiration from Dr. Sherrie Allen)

Faced with any negative situation, ask, "What's in me that's causing this situation to take place, this person to behave this way, this sickness to manifest, this result to be?" Then I say the following four phrases below.

FOUR FUNDAMENTAL HO'OPONOPONO PHRASES

1 - I am sorry.

The moment you take responsibility for negative experiences, you create an opportunity for healing. The apology acknowledges that you are sorry for whatever you or your ancestors have done to cause the negative situation. The apology isn't directed to anyone. Simply say, "I'm sorry."

2 - Please forgive me.

You're asking forgiveness for having attracted the negative situation to your life, missing out on the wonderful experiences you could have had, and complete certainty that it's done. It's essential to know that practitioners never have to forgive anyone because they realize that all wrongdoing came from their actions or memories. Say, "Please forgive me."

3 - I love you.

There is no doubt that love is a powerful healer. When you send unconditional, or agape love through your spirit, it will provide you with an immediate sense of wellbeing. Furthermore, the act of thinking loving thoughts may tune your mind to frequencies possessing incredible and immediate outcomes. I've been told that LOVE is the only force transforming an enemy into a friend. As often as needed, repeat, "I love you."

4 - Thank you.

The moment you take responsibility for the situation, you're guaranteed a response. It may not be what you expect or want. It's your opportunity to start the healing process. You're acknowledging your request was heard and acted on. Simply say, "Thank you."

Important: Never blame others because the problem may reoccur. It won't make you feel better, or start the healing and cleaning process within.

Then, I say, "I'm sorry. Please forgive me. I love you. Thank you." Also, you may say these four phrases after mantras, prayers, and whenever needed.

MY HO'OPONOPONO EXERCISES

Morrnah's Prayer

(Source: Dr. Hew Len, Practitioner)
(I call it forgiveness and healing prayer)

"Spirit, Superconscious, please locate the origin of my memories, beliefs, feelings, thoughts
of:_____.
(Fill in your beliefs, thoughts, and feelings on the line)

Take every level, layer, area, and aspect of my being to these origins. Analyze it and resolve it perfectly with God's truth. Come through all generations of time and eternity–healing every incident and its appendages based on the origin. Please do it according to God's will until I'm at the present, filled with light and truth. God's peace and love, forgiveness of myself for my incorrect perceptions, forgiveness of every person, place, circumstance, and event that contributed to this, these feelings and thoughts.

I'm sorry.
Please forgive me.
I love you.
Thank you."

Take as many deep breaths as you desire. Then hold and release when you're ready. It calibrates your immune system to accept what you stated, according to Dr. Michael Bernard Beckwith's practice at Agape International Spiritual Center.

MY PERSONAL HO'OPONOPONO PRAYERS

I take 100 percent responsibility for whatever problems are within me and everyone in the world and would like you to convert whatever: <u>bad memory, data, and information, health, debt, business, financial, enemy, and relationship blocks and errors to nothing.</u>

Note: the underlined words are examples.

MORRNAH'S PRAYER by Morrnah Simeona

(Forgiveness Prayer)

"Divine creator, father, mother, son as one. If my family, relatives and ancestors, and I have offended you, your family, relatives and ancestors in thoughts, words, deeds and actions from the beginning of our creation to the present, we ask your forgiveness. Let this cleanse, purify, release, cut all the negative memories, blocks, energies and vibrations, and transmute these unwanted energies to pure light. And it is done."

MY PERSONAL HO'OPONOPONO CLEANING LIST

It includes names of people, places, and/or businesses and property addresses that I want God to clean or make right. For example: family members and friends.

To end the practice, I say, "And it is done." Then I take one or as many deep breaths as I desire, hold it, and release it when I'm ready.

Note: After the first year of saying them separately, I've included my Ho'oponopono Cleaning list names of people and things, and addresses at the end of this amazing prayer. For instance, now I say it this way: Let this cleanse, purify, release, cut all the negative memories, blocks, energies and vibrations and transmute these unwanted energies to pure light for me, Althea Moses...

And it is done. I'm sorry. Please forgive me. I love you. Thank you.

It is a man's own mind, not his enemy or foe, that lures him to evil ways. -The Buddha.

MY PERSONAL ADVANCED HO'OPONOPONO MEDITATION

(Inspired by video, Advanced Inner Child Meditation, by Mark Ryan)

With my personal Advanced Ho'oponopono Meditation, I exercise my mind and spirit, for ten minutes daily. In this exercise, I silently talk to my subconscious. I call it Inner Child or Little Althea. According to Dr. Len, this is the place where all of our bad memories, data, and information are stored. To heal ourselves, we must communicate with our subconscious to release or let them go to the Divine God and replace with divine inspirations and guidance from Him.

In reality, this amazing meditation is about ten minutes long. I recommend viewing it in its entirety on YouTube. Below are some of the statements from the beginning of my daily meditation. Each day some of the statements may change.

DESCRIPTION OF MY HO'OPONOPONO MEDITATION

I start with my eyes closed, sitting upright with my feet on the floor and my first and second (on both hands) fingers connected like a chain and placed on my thighs, close to my knees. I start off with a few deep breaths to calm my firm-body temple. I visualize seeing myself as little Althea with a beautiful smile.

Good morning Little Althea. I acknowledge your presence in me. Thank you for being apart of me.

May I please stroke the top of your head with love? I wait for her answer. [Then I stroke the top of her head]

Thank you for being apart of me. I'm sorry for all the bad memories and data you have stored due to my pains and sorrows. Please forgive me. I'm sorry. I love you. Thank you.

I know that you're not the problems I have. I know it's the bad memories and data replaying. I need your help to release these problems. So, please let go of all of them and let the Divine now.

I need you to let go of them so that the Divine can bring us back to zero, make us bad memories, and data free, and we can walk hand in hand into the light with the Divine forevermore. Please help me heal. Thank you. I love you.

Little Althea, please let go of all the bad memories and data replaying as these feelings in my body. Let the Divine now. Thank you. I love you.

Little Althea, can I please hug and show you my love? [I visualize my Inner Child hugging me too.]

Little Althea, I'm sorry for all the stored bad memories and data you have from my pains and sorrows. Please forgive me. I love you. Thank you. I'm glad you're apart of me.

Little Althea, can I please hold and stroke one of your hands with love? [I visualize stroking her hand] What's going on in me that I experienced problems with <u>name person or people</u>. Please let go of the bad memories replaying as these problems with them. Please let go to and let the Divine now. Thank you.

NOTE: I shortened this meditation for time purposes.

Then I take a deep breath, hold it, count to seven, then exhale and count to seven as I rest. I repeat this process six more times.

After two years, my Inner Child embraces me tightly, like she hadn't seen me in a long time. Her unconditional love and cherishing make my eyes well up with tears of joy, and I sigh with a grateful, fulfilled breath.

HEART MEDITATION

(Inspired by Diana Vela)

You've probably heard people say, "My heart said..."
I've been listening to my heart through Heart Meditation. It's powerful and allows connection with my heart.

First, I acknowledge my heart. "I appreciate you being a part of me." I ask my heart to help solve certain things in my personal, business, and recreational life. Then I listen and wait to hear the answers.

Most mornings I hear the answers of my heart and they bring tears of joy to my eyes. For example, I asked my heart, "What am I to do today to bring my book project into reality?" It said, "Just write from your heart and make the words your own."

My tears welled up in my eyes and I immediately took action and started writing this book in 2012—and finished in 2013.

Remember, the heart is filled with love, compassion, grace, wisdom, and authenticity. Be connected with yours and enjoy its benefits.

JOURNALING

After meditations and affirmations, I write in my journal. For more than a decade, I start with, "Good morning, Abba, Jesus, Holy Spirit, and Little Althea. I give thanks and praise. Please forgive us, for we're so lost sometimes. I love you!" Those last three sentences are very similar to the four Ho'oponopono phrases.

"Thank you for your grace, mercies, love, power, protection, healing, and fruits of the Spirit." I also thank God for specific blessings I received that week or whatever is in my heart.

Next, "God, no one loves, protects, heals, comforts, and provides for us as you do." I ask for my heart's desires, wisdom, knowledge, and understanding to keep, handle, and enjoy my blessings. Finally, I thank God for my future blessings. Then I take and hold a deep breath.

Then I close my eyes, ask God, Jesus, and the Holy Spirit to speak to me through their Word. I take my pen, circle it in the air three times, and push it between my Bible pages to open it and choose the Word of the day. I usually read both pages and focus on the underlined words (commonly known as God's words). Most days, the Word I read had a connection with what was going on in my life, or what I've asked the Divine about. I write it on the bottom of my journal page for that day and close with this prayer, "I've hidden your Word in my heart that I may not sin against you, but do your will and intention for my life. Amen.

Scripture I Say at Night

He who dwells in the shelter of the Most High will rest in the shadow of the Almighty...

With long life will I satisfy him and show him my salvation. (Psalm 91 NIV Bible)

You now have many simple and effective practices to incorporate along with what you're already doing to strengthen your mind, spirit, and soul. As you embark on your journey to become irresistibly fit, write down your goals, and be conscious of them. Create a dream board filled with images and words of the things you desire. Ask the Creator to grant you your desires. You're not alone. Never give up. I'm holding a space for you to have success.

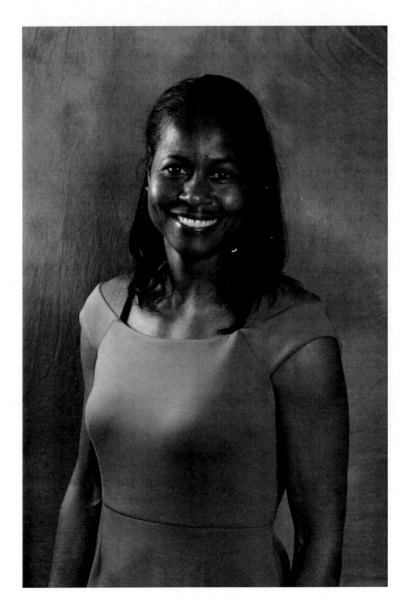

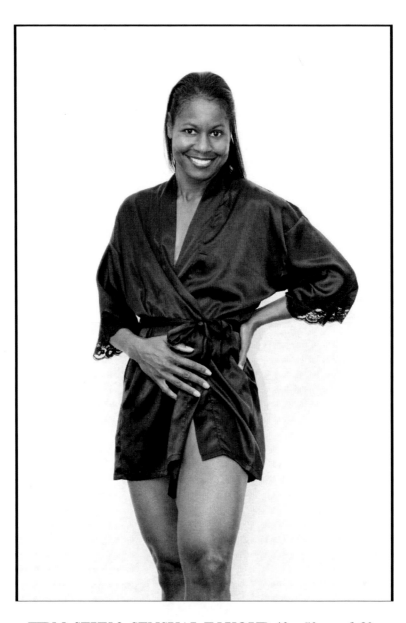

FIRM, SEXY & SENSUAL IN YOUR 40s, 50s, and 60s
YOUR GIFT FROM THE CREATOR

CHAPTER 3

HOW TO BUILD YOUR BODY TEMPLE

A firm-body temple is your perfectly toned, shaped, sexy, sensual, firm, and rock solid sanctuary. It's the body you've been blessed with by your Creator God. According to the Bible, the body is the temple of the living God and the Holy Spirit. Be grateful for the gift of your body temple, which is like no other in the world. Your body temple mold was broken upon your birth. You should honor the Creator God, and yourself with it—not like the world expects you to honor Him.

Your body temple is surely not inferior to someone else's attributes. The Creator God didn't make any mistakes with your body temple. I accept mine and appreciate it in all its uniqueness. It has been freeing to do so. Everyday, you should say, "I love, accept, and appreciate my body temple." You can always use the exercises in this book to improve your body temple. Do it today. What do you have to lose?

I remember, as a freshman in high school, I disliked how my skinny body looked. I started running and lifting weights few times per week. Weeks later, I liked how my body felt and looked. I changed my mindset and language. I affirmed, "I love my body."

I enjoyed seeing how toned, fit, strong, sexy, and sensual it became. Year after year, I kept running, jumping, and lifting weights. When I was unable to lift weights, I did calisthenics. Calisthenics is when you use your body weight to execute exercises like push-ups, squat, calf raises, pull-ups, and sit-ups. Hence, you can do the same, and get great strength and toning results.

After my third Olympic Games competition and more than a decade of running, jumping, and weight training, I was tired of exercising. At age 26, my body was fit, firm, strong, sensual, and sexy. I decided that I didn't need to exercise anymore. Since I was young, I felt that my body wouldn't get out of shape until I reached age forty.

For one year, I didn't exercise like I did for track and field. I walked with no intention to stay in shape.

I felt I had deprived myself of consuming a lot of junk foods, and drinking sugary beverages in the previous decade. For a year, I consumed junk as often as I desired. I was happy!

One day I looked at my body temple in the mirror, and was surprised at its transformation! My legs, arms, back, shoulders, stomach, and buttocks were unfit, unsexy, and not firm. For the first time since my freshman year in high school, my body temple looked unappealing to me. I disliked how my muscles felt soft like marshmallows. I was uncomfortable viewing indentations on my upper back caused by my bra straps. Worse than that, I didn't feel as strong as I did—before track retirement after the Olympic Games.

I made a commitment to live an active lifestyle. I'd execute cardiovascular and strength (weight-lifting) training two to three days per week for the rest of my life. Within few months, my muscles remembered my thirteen years of work and responded with a strong, firm, sensual, and sexy-body temple. Since then, I'm happy with what I see in my mirror, images, and how I feel.

I've been running and weight training for the last couple decades, except for a couple of times after surgery for my Achilles tendon rupture and two major surgeries to remove numerous fibroids from my uterus.

My passion, love of exercise, and the importance of exercising my firm-body temple are known by many people. In the new millennium, after the surgeries, I asked one of my doctors (Dr. Mba) how he felt about me exercising if I felt better. He firmly stated, "You must not exercise for six weeks because your body needs to heal. You need healthy nutrition too." I followed his instructions, but couldn't wait for the day I was released to exercise. When the day came, I was happy to jog, run, and weight train again.

If you dislike the way your body temple looks, sags and feel like marshmallows, use the exercises and nutrition information in this book. You'll start building your body temple to become strong and firm. If you're already building your body temple, use this book to save time by working out two days per week, and maintaining it for life.

Although your body temple looks different from other women, have a great sense of self. Love yourself. Define yourself for yourself. Be happy with the wonderful person you are. Whether or not your body temple is shaped like some famous women in the world (Oprah, Michelle Obama, Beyonce, Angelina Jolei, Ayumi Hamasaki, Kim Kardasian, Coco Lee, Shakira, Jennifer Lopez, Palak Muchhal, Candi Lawrence or mine), you will become sexy and firm by executing the exercises in this book. Then everyone will admire you, and no one can resist you.

Audre Lorde, author and poet wrote, "If I didn't define myself for myself, I would be crunched into other people's fantasies for me and eaten alive."

Lorde and I aren't the only women who feel this way. Lenda Murray, eight-time Ms. Olympia champion explained that she gets off on being a woman, strong, ladylike, and different. You choose and exercise your own approach. Ladylike works for me, and for my firm-body temple clients, too. We're happy and love ourselves—the unique emanations of the Creator God.

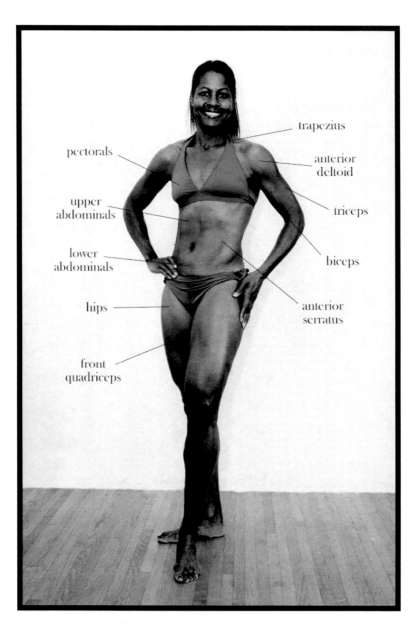

pectorals

trapezius

anterior
deltoid

upper
abdominals

triceps

lower
abdominals

biceps

hips

anterior
serratus

front
quadriceps

A FIRM-BODY TEMPLE

A kind, observant woman complimented me, in a Los Angeles gym. She said, "Excuse me. You have a beautiful back."

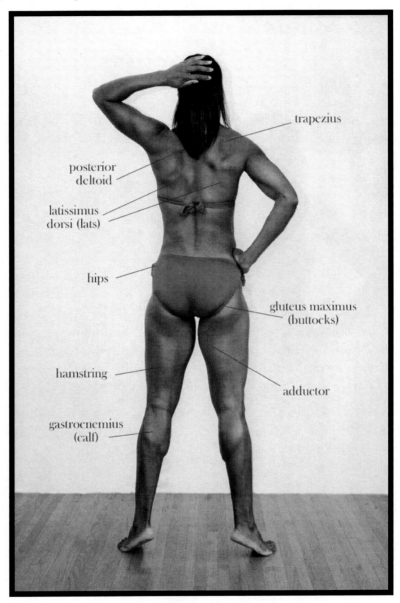

trapezius

posterior deltoid

latissimus dorsi (lats)

hips

gluteus maximus (buttocks)

hamstring

adductor

gastrocnemius (calf)

A FIRM-BODY TEMPLE

CHAPTER 4

BASIC KNOWLEDGE ABOUT YOUR BODY TEMPLE

Your firm-body temple exercises are designed to work on specific muscles. Here are some basic terms about the eight muscle groups on your body. Each one is called a body part. See my images displaying muscle groups on the previous pages.

CHEST

The *chest* muscle is positioned in your breast area. These muscles are called *pectorals*. They help you to move your upper arms.

SERRATUS ANTERIOR and INTERCOSTAL

Serratus anterior and *intercostal* are a common muscle groups not discussed or focused on much, but are admired. *Serratus* are small muscles on your ribs. They can be seen (in front) when you raise your arms, but more likely to be seen if that part is lean.

Intercostal muscles are between your ribs. If you perform them properly, it usually works more muscle groups simultaneously than any other compound exercise for the upper body.

BACK

The *back* is opposite of your chest. Many small muscles are in your back. Two are called *teres major* and *latissimi dorsi,* or "lats." You'll develop the small muscles, then the "lats" and each trapezius muscle.

SHOULDERS

The *shoulders* have two muscles—the *deltoids* and *trapezii*. *Deltoids* are positioned in the front and rear shoulders. The *trapezii* are positioned between your neck and shoulder on each side of your upper back.

ABDOMINALS (ABS)

Rectus Abdominis muscles (commonly called a*bdominals* abdomen, stomach, or "abs"*)* are positioned between your breast and upper thighs. They play a role in maintaining posture.

Note: If you have excess fat on your abdomen or chest (torso), you need to burn more calories with cardio and abdominal exercises, and change to a lean protein, low-calorie and low-fat diet. If you don't change your diet and perform cardio exercises, the fat will prevent you from gracing your eyes on your hardworking, shapely stomach and chest muscles. For example, when some of my clients failed to follow recommendations to tone abs, they experienced frustration and disappointment. Why? They're doing crunches every workout, but not seeing results. To get optimal results with their abs, they needed to change their diet to lean protein, low calories and low fat, and perform cardio and abdominal exercise two to three days per week.

BICEPS

Bicep muscles are on the front of the upper arms between shoulders and elbows. It's the muscle (the size of a small orange or large grapefruit) that many people display when asked to show off their muscle. Arnold Schwarzenegger, Lee Haney, Ronnie Coleman, Rachel McLish, Kim Chizevsky, Iris Kyle, and Lenda Murray displayed their biceps to win the Mr. Olympia or Ms. Olympia bodybuilding titles.

TRICEPS

Triceps are the muscles between your elbows and armpits, positioned on the opposite side each of your biceps. On many out-of-shape middle-aged and elderly men and women, the triceps hang or sag, like a turkey′s neck.

LEGS (CALVES, QUADRICEPS, ADDUCTORS, and HAMSTRINGS)

The muscles of the *legs* are calves, *quadriceps*, *adductors*, and *hamstrings*. The *calf* is the rear-lower half of the leg. They're usually developed in women who run a lot and/or wear high-heeled shoes daily. The *quadriceps* (thighs) are the front muscles between the hip and knee. The *hip-joint adductors* muscles work to pull the legs toward the midline of your body temple. The *hamstrings* are the rear muscles between the buttocks and knees.

BUTTOCKS (GLUTEUS MAXIMUS)

The *buttocks* are the largest muscles in your body. They're above the upper legs in the rear, start in your back hipbone, and run to your tailbone. These muscles are called *gluteus maximus*. When they're developed, the buttocks are coveted by men and women. Some people call them "round buttocks," "apple bottoms," or "onions." As we age and/or become inactive, they start to sag and have unsightly fat (known as "cellulite") all over. As we age, cellulite is more visible on some women's body temple because the skin gets thin.

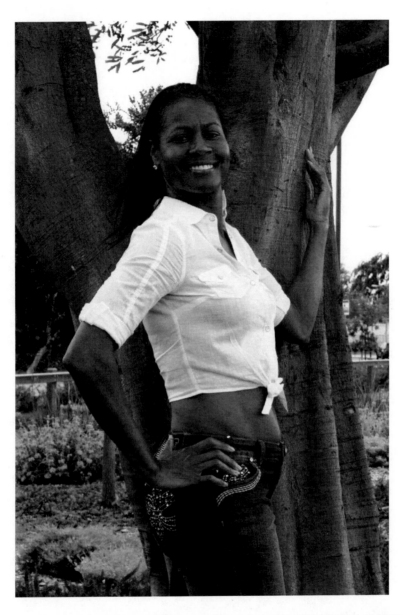

A TONED, STRONG, FIT BODY TEMPLE IS YOUR GIFT.

I believe you can maximize every amount of potential. Decide to do it for yourself. -Althea Moses

CHAPTER 5

BASIC PRINCIPLES AND TERMS

It's important to know the basic principles and terms to be able to use controlled weights to build your firm-body temple effectively and safely. This chapter will explain some of the basic principles and terms.

BASIC AND ISOLATION EXERCISES

Basic exercises work your large muscles. They're done with relatively heavy weights. For example, a basic exercise for quadriceps and hamstrings is the leg press. The weight of the leg press needs to be at least thirty pounds to be effective--even for a weak individual.

Isolation exercises work smaller muscles and are done with relatively lighter weight. For example, an isolation exercise for your upper legs is *leg curl*. This exercise works the hamstrings. It can be done on a leg-curl bench with light weights. You can do one-legged or double-legged curls. A weak individual can use a ten-pound weight. This may be equivalent to 30 pound weights used to do squats.

Another example is the squat—exercise stresses the whole area of the front and rear upper legs, abdominals, buttocks, obliques, and abductors. The leg extension stresses the quadriceps. This Firm-Body Temple workout will provide you with the correct balance of basic and isolation exercises.

DEFINITION

EXERCISE

Exercise is any activity or group of movements being performed to improve or maintain physical fitness and wellness. For example, *ALTHEA*, arm curls, brisk walking, and running.

REPETITION OR REP

Repetition or *rep* is a complete movement of an exercise from where you started to the midpoint and back to where you started. Depending on your fitness and strength level, you should perform eight to twelve repetitions per set, per body part. For instance, in the leg raises exercise, a rep is from where you raised upward to your toes and lowered your heal back to where you started on the floor.

If you choose to do modified pyramiding, perform twelve to fifteen reps on your first set, eight to ten reps on your second set, and six to eight reps on the third set. Most professional bodybuilders perform up to fifteen repetitions.

REST

Pausing, or not working between sets is called *rest*. Couple minutes are good to rest between reps. Rest is essential because muscles attain strength to perform with maximized effort.

SET

A *set* is a group of repetitions. Perform sets and rest in between for one to two minutes. Three sets of an exercise is usually enough to build strong, firm, sexy, and sensual muscles.

If you want to really challenge your muscles, perform four sets of exercise per body part. Lift heavy weights with low reps--your muscles will grow.

ROUTINE

A *routine* is a series of different exercises that are performed with a certain amount of sets. In many cases your workout will include three sets of exercises per body part or nine sets of exercises called your *routine*.

DEFINITION

Definition is when your muscle is clearly visible due to absence of excess body fat. Veins and striations are usually visible. Definition is achieved by performing many repetitions as body fat melts away—lean protein, a low-fat diet, and healthy water may help too.

FREE WEIGHTS (Dumbbells and Barbells)

Dumbbells and *barbells* are called *free weights* because they aren't fixed to the floor and can be carried around. They force you to perform all the work. Most dumbbells and barbell plates have the poundage written on them.

A *dumbbell* is a short bar with a weight at each end, and used to exercise one to two arms at time. A b*arbell* is a long metal bar with disks (plates) of different weights attached at each end. Multiple disks can be added and held in place with devices called *collars.* Some barbells have weights permanently connected for efficiency.

HEAVY VS LIGHT

It's essential to use the *heavy* vs *light* principle if your goal is to build a firm-body temple. Very thin people who want to gain muscle mass, need to lift heavy weights with low repetitions, or reps. People who want to decrease their size, remove excess fat, and shape their body temple need to lift light weights with high repetitions. Those who aren't thin or with excess fat will use a combination of heavy and light weights to achieve their firm-body temple goals.

Heavy weights and low repetitions build mass, and light weights and high repetitions decrease size and give tone or shape.

MACHINES (EQUIPMENT)

Most gyms have a variety of *machines,* or *equipment* to exercise muscles. Many brand-named machines are available, but that doesn't matter because most of your body temple exercises will be done with free weights.

Some machines operate on pulleys, while others operate on cams (curved wheels mounted on rotating shafts). They take some of the stress away from you and cause you to cheat. Machines can be used for variety.

POWER CORDS

The firm-body temple program uses mostly dumbbells, but power cards can be used for variety, or when you're unable to use dumbbells to perform strength or resistance training.

Power cords (resistance bands) are large, lightweight elastic or rubber bands pulled to create resistance to exercise your body parts. Pack them in your purse, tote, or suitcase, and take them anywhere. Varied shapes, resistance levels, and sizes are available at stores.

For example, they might be tubular with handles, or lengths of flat elastic material. My personal preference is the tube-shaped cords with handles.

The benefits of power cords are: increased muscle strength, size, and toning, and more calories burning--leads to fat or weight loss. They keep tension throughout the full range of motion of your exercises.

Power cords work many parts of a lift that aren't often done by free weights. They help to increase flexibility and strength.

Everyone can benefit from using power cords. That includes the elderly because it takes pressure off joints while increasing strength and flexibility. For active individuals and athletes, it's a great addition to get a bigger *pump* from your workout.

If you're a beginning user of power cords, start with the lowest resistance level, and move up as your muscles become stronger. Many of my clients said they anticipated that power cords would be easier to use than lifting dumbbells and barbells. They were surprised to find it's not as easy as it looks.

PROGRESSION

Progression is the gradual and continual adding of weights to your sets to make your muscles work harder. This can be done over a course of weeks or months.

When the muscles work harder, they grow in size and density, becoming shapelier, firmer, and sexier.

As time progresses, you'll find that some of your sets become easier. Increase the weights to make the muscle continue to work and grow.

PUMP

Pump is when your expanded muscle feels the rush of the blood moving through it due to the intense movement of your reps. For instance, when your shoulder muscles seem enlarged after your shoulder routine, it's pumped!

SLEEP AND REST

Your muscles need s*leep* and *rest* to repair and grow. They need time to release the waste products, which were produced from your workout and refuel your muscles with oxygen and glycogen (type of sugar). Your body temple needs about six to eight hours of sleep to make your muscles grow and allow you to concentrate for your next workout session.

SPLIT ROUTINE

The *split routine* is when you allow your muscles to rest for a day before working them again. This is essential for repairing and growing—especially if you want to build a firm-body temple. The split routine ensures that muscles grow to your desired size without compromising energy and unproductive effort.

For example, if you've worked your legs, biceps, and triceps on Wednesday, then you'll work your back, chest, and shoulders on Thursday. You can work abdominals daily.

TRAINING PARTNER

Training partner is a person who motivates, works out with and assists you. *Irresistibly Fit* and I are your official-training partners. Partner with me to become your personal coach and consultant. Take this book to each workout session. If you're in the gym and need a *spotter* (someone to help with weights), ask for help.

VISUALIZATION AND CONCENTRATION

I believe that *visualizing* what you want your body temple to look like while lifting weights can significantly help your body temple become sexy and firm. I used this technique when I was on and off the track. It worked well for me.

Use your mind to concentrate on the parts of your body that you want to change. Imagine excess fat melting from you arms, hips, legs, buttocks, and stomach as you get pumped on each set. Picture yourself in a swimsuit with your firm-body temple looking sexy and sensual.

Tell your muscles to grow and be shapely as you desire. They'll do just that with the use of this book, visualization, concentration, and hard work.

WORKOUT

Your total firm-body temple building session for a given day is called a *workout*. It includes every set you completed for all the body parts you worked. The word *work*, in *workout*, means to challenge your muscles to the maximum. Let's get to work!

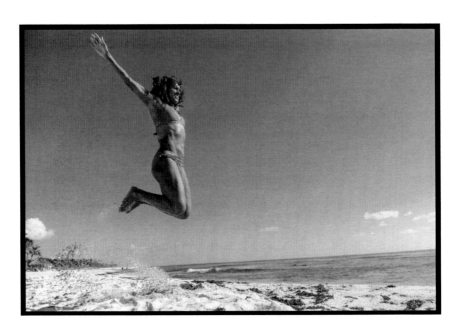

LIVING AN ACTIVE LIFESTYLE WILL MAKE YOU IRRESISTIBLY FIT

Two of the basic requirements for a healthy and happy life are fresh air and exercise, to which the benefit of sunlight exposure is also added. If we were smart, we would view exercise as crucial to our survival. -Rita Elkins

CHAPTER 6

ELEMENTS OF FITNESS AND HOW TO IMPROVE IT

CARDIOVASCULAR CAPACITY (also AEROBIC FITNESS) is the capacity of your heart and lungs, and their system of blood vessels to provide oxygen and nutrients to your body temple. It enables you to run, swim, skate, walk, bike, ski, golf, and dance farther and longer, and with less effort than before. Good conditioning lowers your risk of several diseases, like heart disease and diabetes.

CARDIOVASCULAR ENDURANCE is aerobic activity performed for a long duration and you're usually having fun doing it. For instance, you can do brisk walking, light, moderate and intense jogging and running, cross-country running and skiing, golfing, dancing, skating, swimming, and playing basketball and soccer.

ANAEROBIC CAPACITY is your stored fuel system for short term and intense activities. It enables you to swim or run short distances rapidly. Remember the *N* in anaerobic means no oxygen.

ANAEROBIC CAPACITY is bursts of intense short duration movements, or activities. Running, sprinting, jump roping, swimming, skipping, bike riding, and tumbling are examples of activities. They'll make you feel like you're out of breath.

HIIT or **High Intensity Interval Training** is an example of workout to test your anaerobic capacity. Perform HIIT by alternating short and hard exertions with less difficult ones. For example, sprint sixty meters, rest sixty meters, then sprint sixty meters again--or run in place. Repeat six to eight times. After the first or second time (interval), you should feel like you're out of breath. The way you feel depends on your fitness level. About five years now, HIIT is what I use for my cardio workout—only four minutes and it's done. Research shows that HIIT and strength training (performed on the same day) help you burn calories one to two days later.

STRENGTH is the ability to move heavy weight at least one or more times. Increasing muscle strength lessens the difficulty of lifting weights and moving your body temple around. Weak muscles can lose functional-lean muscle mass and cause physical health problems. For instance, weak quadriceps increases the risk of knee injury and arthritis.

STRENGTH - Build strength from using weights, power cords, and your body weight (calisthenics). It's useful for getting up and down from the floor, push-ups and pull-ups, lifting furniture, and doing other fun, functional, body exercises.

For teens and most adults, slowly and safely lift the heaviest weight you can lift for 8 to 12 times. Complete three sets.

Elderly people can build strength by lifting the heaviest weight four to eight times. The more you lift that weight, the stronger your muscles will become, and you'll be able to increase the weight amount.

POWER is the ability to use physical force to move weight, or your body quickly. You need and use power to throw, pull, push, punch, and lift.

POWER - safely lift or move a heavy weight, power cord (s), your body, or light object quickly. Repeat as many times as possible. For example, use a power cord to do bicep curls, side lateral raises, one arm triceps extension, and standing glute-kickback.

MUSCULAR ENDURANCE is ability to support or move a weight repeatedly. For example, muscular endurance of your legs is necessary to walk and jog, run, dance, and bike ride long distances. Your shoulders and torso use muscular endurance to stand and sit in a healthy position, like when you're watching television and reading a book.

MUSCULAR ENDURANCE - safely perform continuous lifting or movements with relatively lighter weights or power cords.

FLEXIBILITY is ability to move your body safely, with ease, through a range of motions.

FLEXIBILITY - Keep your back upright when sitting and standing to prevent you from slouching (over stretching and rounding it). To prevent serious back injury, always bend your knees from a standing position to pick up things or children. Slowly stretch muscles (daily) to maintain your ability to stand straight and move or flex in healthy ways. Don't bounce when stretching. You can use power cords to improve flexibility and achieve great returns for your time and effort.

BALANCE is the ability to keep your body temple steady to keep from slipping, swinging, wobbling, or falling. Your balance may be impacted by diseases, injuries, and lack of muscle use--sedentary lifestyle.

BALANCE - It's beneficial for independence, ease of movement with your varied activities, and prevention of sprains and falls. Some easy things to build balance include: putting on and taking off your socks, shoes, and pants, and standing on one foot as you brush your teeth, wash dishes, comb your hair, and talk on the telephone.

MENTAL FITNESS is performed by your mind. This includes pattern recognition, memorization, problem solving, and other thinking functions. With regular practice, your mental fitness will and/or can improve function at any age.

MENTAL FITNESS - Exercise or practice your mental abilities, daily, to keep them functioning at any age. For example: painting, sculpting, drawing, learning a new language, practicing with musical instruments, building something, solving problems, and teaching others your favorite skill. Problem solving, pattern recognition, and puzzle games on your smartphone, iPad, and laptop computer also increase mental fitness.

EMOTIONAL FITNESS pertains to a healthy or fit brain strengthened with regular exercise of the mind and body. Several sections of your brain that process self-control help improve emotional fitness. An essential part of self-control is refraining from harmful actions and thoughts, and engaging in positive ones. For example, don't harm yourself with bad decisions, or negative thoughts.

EMOTIONAL FITNESS - Essential parts of the emotional fitness element are refraining from habit forming, unhealthy harmful actions and thoughts, and engaging in good thoughts and actions. Exercise positive thoughts and actions that'll bring forth positive actions like kindness, self-discipline, goodness, faithfulness, and happiness. Say affirmations: "I love you. I'm loved. I'm love. I'm special. I'm powerful. I'm strong. I'm worthy. I'm enough. I'm good. I'm sorry. I forgive you."

SIZE - Build muscle size by lifting moderate to heavy weights with less repetition, two times per week. Along with strength and/or weight training exercises, consume low fat and high protein foods (or whey protein) to repair and make muscles grow. Protein ignites your fat burning hormones too. (Details in the Nutritional Choices chapter).

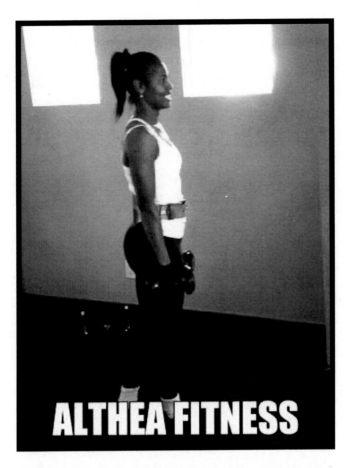

I'M DETERMINED TO REMAIN STRONG.

A firm-body temple builder, without effective workout tools and
fuel, is set to fail.
-Althea Moses

CHAPTER 7

BASIC WORKOUT TOOLS AND FUEL

These tools are recommendations to assist you in having a comfortable, safe experience during your firm-body temple workouts.

- Comfortable walking, running, or cross-training shoes
- Pair of workout gloves to protect your hands
- Workout belt to protect back (heavy weightlifters)
- Workout towel
- Sets of dumbbells and power cords (5, 10, 15 lb)
- Sets of ankle weights
- *Irresistibly Fit Workbook* to record your progress and successes and more
- Exercise mat
- Gym bag

HIGHLY RECOMMENDED: Alkaline water with added hydrogen.

Alkaline water helps with quicker cellular absorption and hydration. Alkaline water with added hydrogen (excellent antioxidant) helps with removal of lactic acid from muscles, toxins from cells, and free radicals.

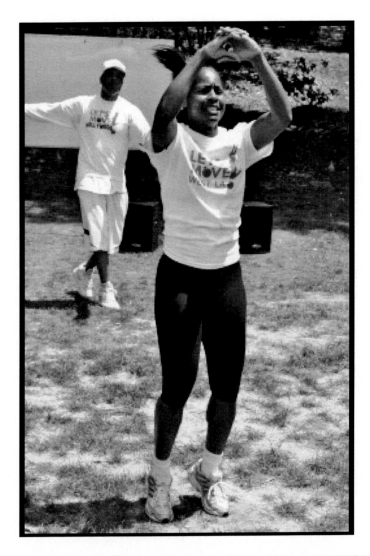

ALTHEA EXERCISE AND CIRCLEMARK MAKE YOU IRRESISTIBLY FIT ™

Keeping the body in good health is a duty. Otherwise the body should not be able to be strong and clear. -Buddha

CHAPTER 8

FIVE TO TEN MINUTE WARM UP

Stretching is not a warm up. You should always warm up your body temple about five to ten minutes. It helps to raise your body temperature, and gets blood and oxygen into your heart and muscles easier. Blood circulation makes your muscles become more pliable and work faster. If you don't warm up, you'll feel tight, work slower, be less flexible and energized, and more important, increase your risk of injuring your muscles.

You don't have to warm up for more than ten minutes to perform cardio or strength training. Choose from a variety of exercises to warm up before stretching your muscles. You're warmed up when you break a light sweat.

After your warm up, stretch your muscles about five to ten minutes. Stretching helps to make your muscles flexible, safe to exercise, and endure more force without excessive tearing or injury.

EXERCISES TO WARM UP: *ALTHEA* technique (exercise), brisk walking, jogging, cycling on a stationary bike, jump roping, dancing, light swimming, and properly executed push-ups, and lunges.

MUSIC TO WARM UP AND WORKOUT

Recent research shows that listening to music while exercising boosted verbal fluency skills and cognitive levels in people diagnosed with coronary artery disease. Music may also increase your endurance and improve your performance by up to twenty percent. Uptempo music can motivate you to run faster even if you're exhausted.

If you enjoy music, I recommend creating a playlist of your favorite songs on a device, like smartphone with headset or earbuds. You'll be motivated and have quality workouts.

I enjoy warming up with uplifting, uptempo, funky bass rhythm songs, like *Stone Love,* written by the late musical genius Kashif and co-writer Lala. Also, I enjoy listening to *Pump it Up* by the legendary singer Lord Rhaburn. My playlist includes music from diverse genres: reggae, soca, punta rock, R&B, and pop.

Recent research found that listening to music causes much more to happen in your body temple than basic auditory processing. Music triggers activity in a part of the brain that releases dopamine—the feel good chemical.

Many active, bodybuilding, and/or athletic individuals agree about the impact of dopamine. For instance, when I listen to *Stone Love,* the music and lyrics excite me about working out and feeling good about loving myself! It sets the tone to experience quality workouts while repeating the affirmation, "I exercise because I love myself." Why do you exercise?

After listening to and singing along with *Stone Love,* on my warm up and stretch sessions, I feel so loved, cherished, and happy! The lyrics remind me that God loves me, I love me, and for me to give love, I must love myself. As a result, I'm smiling, dancing, and pumping weights with a lot of energy and strength during my workout sessions.

Sometimes, I listen to the Rocky movie songs, *Going the Distance* and *No Easy Way Out,* written by Bill Conti. The titles of those songs illustrate what I believe I need to do and remember as I maintain my firm-body temple.

I've found that listening to music during my workout motivates me to perform my best, and have much fun. Music makes my workouts feel shorter than they really were.

WARM UP PROGRAM INTRODUCTION

ALTHEA Technique (Exercise)

Brisk Walking or Light Jogging

Jump Roping

Cycling on Stationary Bike

Cycling on exercise mat, or carpeted floor with legs only

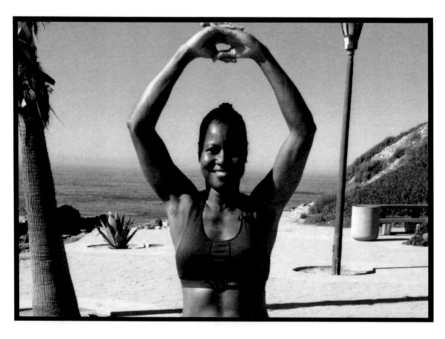

ALTHEA EXERCISE AND CIRCLEMARK MAKE YOU IRRESISTIBLY FIT

ALTHEA

(Warm up exercise with Circlemark hand gesture)

This exercise will raise your body temperature, and enhance your self-awareness to acceptance of wholesomeness, power, sacred space, and love.

PREPARATION/DIRECTIONS

⇒ Stand in neutral position with arms to your sides.

⇒ Gently clasp your fingers together; position slightly away from your chest. Hold.

⇒ Keep your elbows touching your sides.

⇒ Position your right thumb under your left thumb to see a circle shape or circle mark.

⇒ Hold up your circle hand gesture slightly away from your chest. Relax.

⇒ Take a deep breath and hold it for seven seconds. Repeat. Smile. Relax.

⇒ Say, "I love you," aloud, or silently as many times as you like.

MOVEMENT

⇒ Hold up your circle hand gesture slightly away from your chest.

⇒ Gently bend your knees, jump, and raise circle hand gesture above your head.

⇒ Continue jumping in place and raising circle hand gesture above your head.

⇒ Repeat as you say, "I love you," aloud, or silently

⇒ Continue full *Althea* movement and phrase. Smile and have fun!

⇒ Perform movement for 5-10 minutes. You're warmed up if you start to sweat.

Note: Sweating may occur depending on your health condition.

VARIATION

Perform this exercise in front a mirror to see your circle hand gesture. Options: jump with both legs forward/backwards/sideways. Jump on one leg, jog in place/forward/backward, move feet outward, kick each leg forward, backward, sideways. Lift each knee to your waist.

If you're unable to jump, jog, or kick, bend knees repeatedly to do short squats.

Say affirmations: I'm wholesome. I'm God's child. I'm powerful. I'm free. I'm beautiful. I'm love. I'm loved. I forgive you. I'm happy. I'm determined to lose weight. I'm well. I'm strong. I'm enough. I'm lovable. I'm determined to get fit. I'm determined to be healthy.

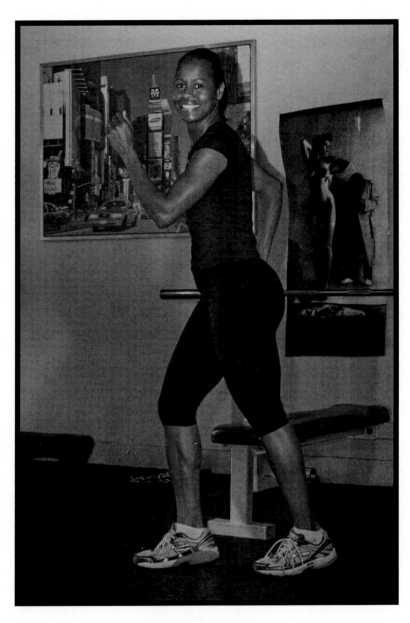

BRISK WALKING

BRISK WALKING

These exercises will raise your body temple's temperature. If you do these exercises for thirty minutes per day, or ten minutes three times per day, three to four times per week, you'll improve your cardiovascular fitness level.

DIRECTIONS

Move your arms and feet quickly—a moderate pace or intensity.

Move your arms to the maximum position in front and behind you.

Remember, it's not your regular pace. It's brisk walking.

VARIATIONS

Move your feet quickly with short or long strides.

You'll cover less distance with short strides.

You'll cover more distance with long strides.

Your pace is good if you're unable to have a comfortable conversation during the exercise.

LIGHT JOGGING

This exercise raises your body temperature.

If you perform this exercise thirty minutes per day, or ten minutes three times per day for three to four times per week, you'll increase your cardiovascular fitness level.

DIRECTIONS

Run at a leisurely slow pace (low intensity).

VARIATIONS

Run at a slightly faster pace with moderate intensity.

Monitor your heart rate by touching your pulse.

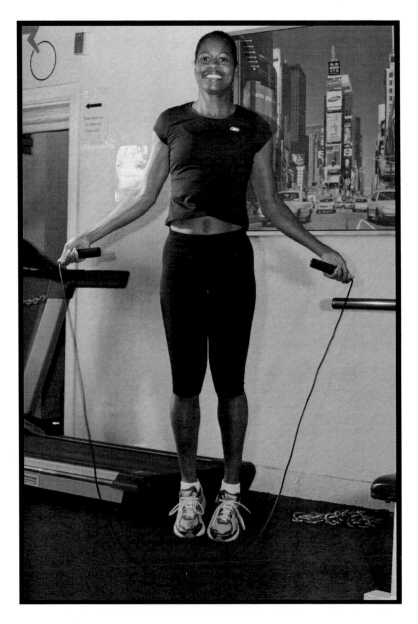

BASIC JUMP ROPING

BASIC JUMP ROPING

This exercise raises your body temple's temperature.
A great exercise to increase your cardio fitness level.

DIRECTIONS

Grasp the jump rope in each hand and extend from your body.
Start with the jump rope behind you on the floor or ground.

MOVEMENT

Swing it slowly from behind you, then over your head to the front of
you and jump over it as it hits the floor or ground.
Repeat slowly to moderately for five minutes without stopping
Note: If you stop before time ends, continue the movement.

VARIATIONS

Perform jump roping like former First Lady Michelle Obama when
she's in a hotel room, or on campaigning trips with her husband and
former President Barack Obama.

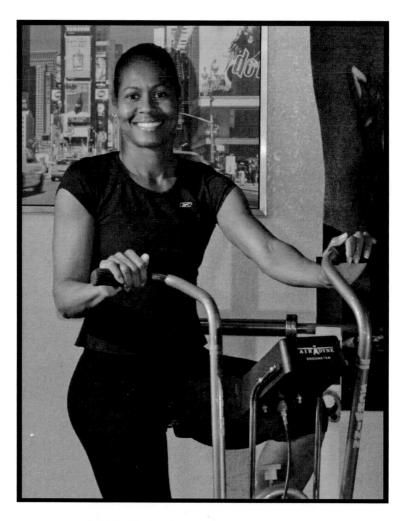

CYCLING ON A STATIONARY BIKE

This exercise raises your body temple's temperature.

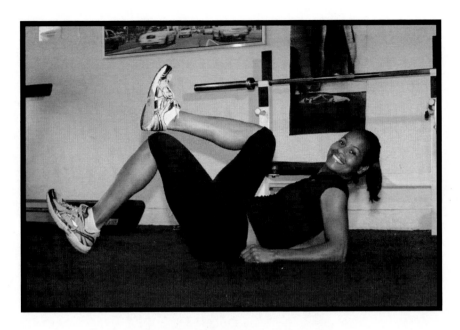

CYCLING WITHOUT A BIKE

CYCLING WITHOUT A BIKE

This exercise raises your body temple's temperature.

DIRECTIONS

Lie on your exercise mat and raise your legs straight up into the air.

Position your hands near your buttocks and raise your hips until your body weight is supported by your shoulders.

Hold your hips upward with your hands.

Keep your elbows still on your exercise mat.

MOVEMENT

Move your legs in a circular movement, as if you were pedaling a bicycle.

Bring your knees near your face as possible.

Be sure to control your movement to protect from hitting your stomach and chest with your knees.

Repeat for a minute for five sets.

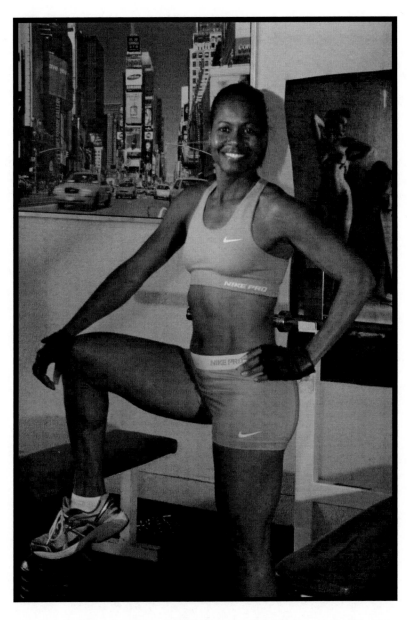

HAPPY, HEALTHY, AND IRRESISTIBLY FIT MODEL

STRETCHING YOUR BODY TEMPLE

When you stretch your muscles, you're lengthening and relaxing them.

Although stretching is not a warm up, it's very important to stretch your muscles after raising your body temple's temperature with one of the exercises in this chapter. In particular, stretching will make your warmed up muscles more pliable, work faster, stretch more, and endure much more force without painful tearing.

Remember to always stretch in a slow controlled way. Hold them to the point of slight discomfort—not pain. NEVER bounce when stretching. Breathe normal. Please don't ever hold your breath.

STRETCHING PROGRAM INTRODUCTION

Neutral Position

Overhead Reach

Side Torso Stretch

Torso and Obliques Stretch

Quadriceps Stretch (Pull leg behind with foot to buttocks)

Hamstrings Stretch (Lift knee to chest and hold)

Hamstrings and Calf Stretch (Lift right leg onto a metal bar for stretching, table, or desk)

Calf Stretch

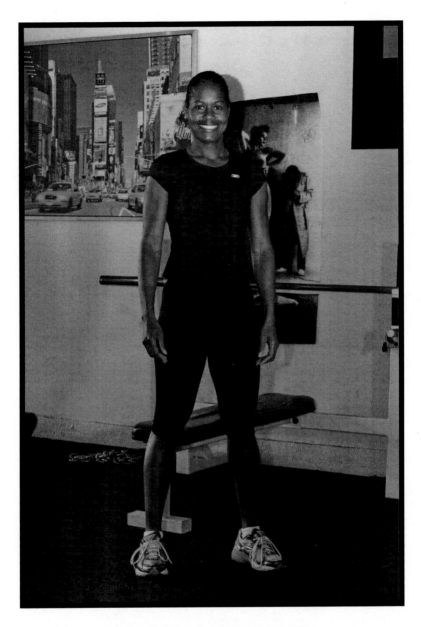

NEUTRAL POSITION STAND

Stand upright with feet shoulder-width apart, and arms to sides.

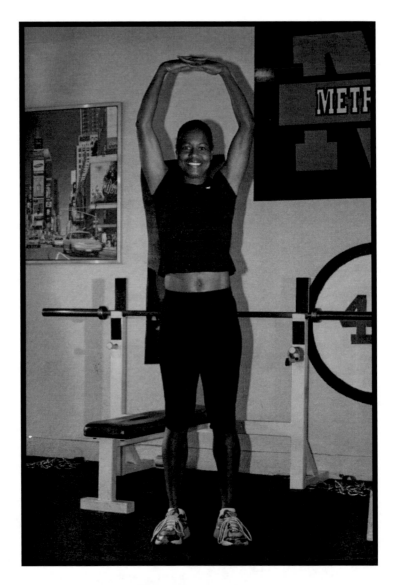

OVERHEAD REACH

This stretch relaxes your shoulders, triceps, and biceps.

Stand in neutral position with feet shoulder width apart. Raise both arms, and reach over your head.

Hold stretch for thirty seconds. Then relax.

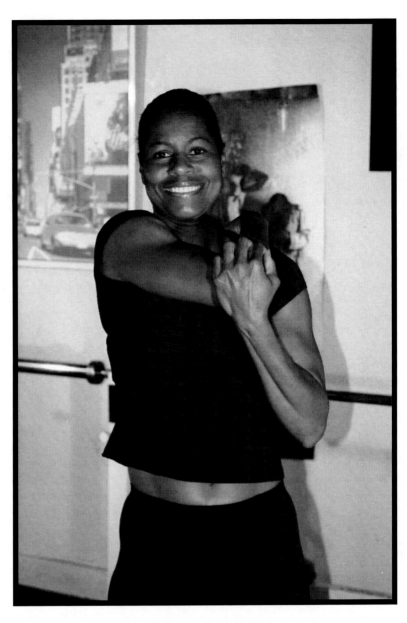

TRICEPS, TORSO, AND BACK STRETCH

TRICEPS, TORSO, AND BACK STRETCH

This stretch relaxes your shoulders, triceps, biceps, and back.

Stand in neutral position with legs shoulder width apart, and knees slightly bent.

Place left hand on right shoulder, and right forearm behind left upper arm.

Pull left arm across chest. Turn torso to the right.

Hold for thirty seconds. Relax.

Do the same exercise with the right hand on the left shoulder.

SIDE-BEND TORSO STRETCH

This stretch relaxes your sides, torso, and waist.

Raise both arms high above your head.

Lock fingers with palms open.

Lean to right side.

Hold stretch for thirty seconds.

Breathe normally during stretch.

Lean to center.

Return to your left.

Hold stretch for thirty seconds.

Return to center and release fingers.

Slowly move your arms to your side.

Relax.

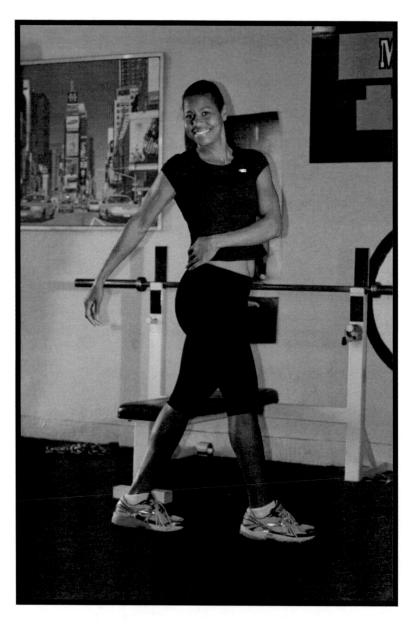

TORSO AND OBLIQUES STRETCH

TORSO AND OBLIQUES STRETCH

This stretch relaxes your torso and *obliques*—side muscles.

Start in a neutral position.

Position right foot twenty-four inches behind the left foot.

Keep your knee slightly bent on the forward leg.

Gently turn body temple toward the forward leg, or left side.

Your right hand holds the hip of the forward or left leg. Hold for thirty seconds.

Return to neutral position. Switch legs.

Position left foot behind right foot.

Repeat the above directions.

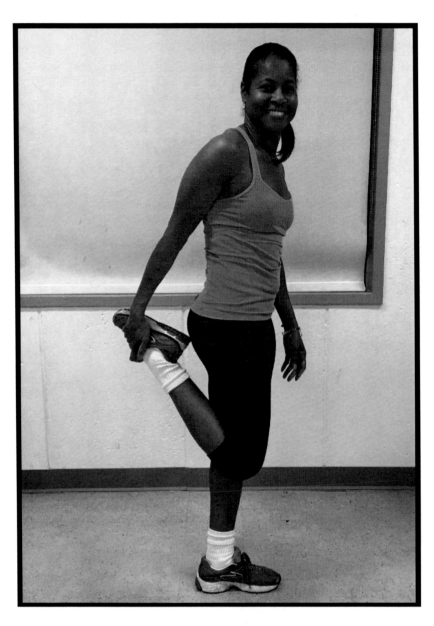

QUADRICEPS STRETCH

QUADRICEPS STRETCH

This stretch relaxes your quadriceps (thigh) muscles.

Start at neutral position with feet shoulder width apart.

Keep back straight.

Keep knees close to together as possible.

Grasp left foot with left hand and pull heel to your buttocks.

Hold for thirty seconds.

NOTE: Raise your right hand high above your head. It helps with balance. Repeat with right foot and right hand.

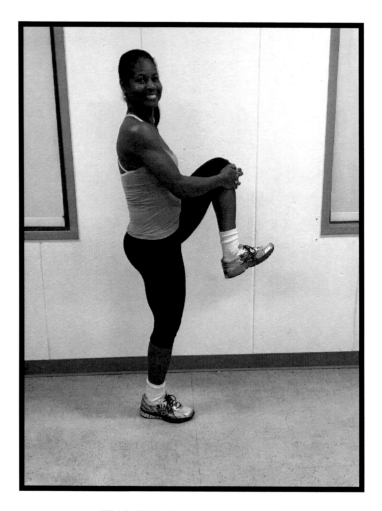

HAMSTRINGS STRETCH

HAMSTRINGS STRETCH

This relaxes the hamstring muscle (rear of upper legs).

Stand in neutral position.

Raise left leg to your hip.

Hold leg with both hands.

Pull leg towards chest with your fingers locked.

Hold for thirty seconds.

Stand in neutral position.

Repeat with right leg.

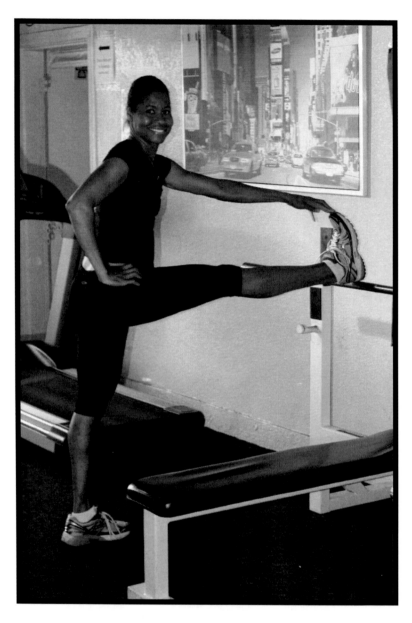

HAMSTRINGS AND CALVES STRETCH

HAMSTRINGS AND CALVES STRETCH

This stretch relaxes your hamstrings and calves.

Stand in neutral position with legs slightly apart.

Raise up left leg and place on a wall or bar, desk, etc.

Hold for thirty seconds.

Keep back straight.

Repeat stretch with right leg.

VARIATION:
LYING DOWN HAMSTRING STRETCH

(This is a great stretch. Keeps your back straight and pressure off the discs.)

Lie down on your back. Raise right leg to your hip.

Keep head, shoulders, and buttocks on the floor.

Keep leg straight upward to the sky for about thirty seconds.

Keep the left leg straight as possible—on the floor. Switch to right leg.

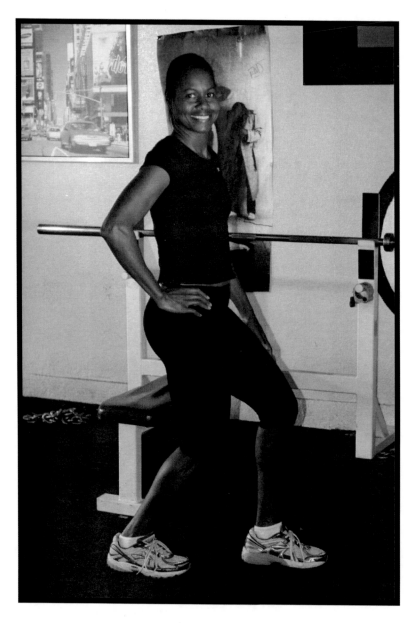

CALVES STRETCH

CALVES STRETCH

This stretch relaxes your calves.

Stand in neutral position.

Step forward about twenty-four inches with your left leg.

Keep back straight.

Bend right knee gently.

Hold stretch for thirty seconds.

Stand in neutral position.

Step forward about twenty-four inches apart with your right leg.

Keep back straight.

Bend left knee gently.

Hold stretch for thirty seconds. Relax.

COOL DOWN (WARM DOWN)

Always cool down (warm down) your muscles by stretching after each workout—about five to ten minutes. It assists in opening circulation to and moving the lactic acid out of your muscles. It prevents tightness, lessens soreness, and risk of injuries.

Perform any of the stretches used to warm up your body temple.

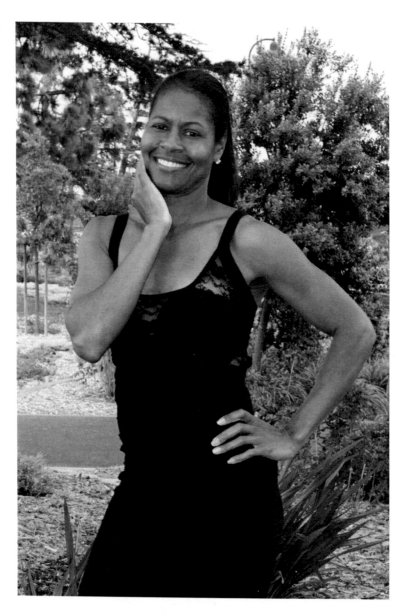

I'M FIT AND WELL.

The sport and lifestyle belie the myths and stereotypes of femininity; the women of bodybuilding are on the cutting edge of cultural change! -Bill Dobbins (body photographer/author)

CHAPTER 9

WORKOUTS FOR THREE BODY-TEMPLE SIZES

Strength and/or weight training improves your endurance, power, strength, and health. These weight-training workouts are for three body temple sizes. I call them *Out-of-Shape*, *Thin*, and *Large*. The *Out-of-Shape* body temple isn't overweight, fat, or fit. *Out-of-Shape* bodies look great in clothes, but not so desirable in a bathing suit. The arms are slightly sagging, and there's cellulite on their hips, buttocks, stomach, back, and legs.

The *Thin* body temple could be underweight and unshapely with little fat, and may want to add mass.

The *Large* body temple could be overweight with excess fat, cellulite on hips, buttocks, arms, and legs. They want to lose the excess fat, and come down in size.

No matter what your size, or fitness level, your goal is to strengthen muscles, and decrease unappealing, spongy, lumpy fat, and replace it with firm, shapely muscles for women, and firm large muscles for men. With strength and weight training, cardiovascular activities, and good food choices, the body parts you worked will lose fat—especially your legs, buttocks, abdominals, back, and triceps. They'll become firm, shapely, sexy, and sensual.

Remember weight training doesn't always mean "bodybuilding." If you choose to perform cardio exercises and skip weight-training exercises, however, you'll be what some health and fitness experts refer to as a "skinny-fat person," —not overweight, but usually lacking firm, sexy, and sensual muscles.

Science states that after your weight-training workouts, your body continues burning calories, and losing fat while you're sleeping, reading, and watching TV. This incredible information keeps me highly motivated to continue strength and weight training.

If your body temple's size is *Large*, it's important to be patient. It may take you longer than the other body types to see shapely, sexy, sensual muscles. With consistency and hard work, you may achieve a firm-body temple in six months to a year.

One female client (*Large* body temple) said, "I'm going to do whatever I need to because I want to bring my sexy back." She took a long time to gain the weight, so she's patient with the process. Hence, it may to take a long time for the weight to come off.

For *Thin* body temples, you'll see shapely, sexy, sensual muscles in about four to six months. The *Out-of-Shape* body temples, you'll see shapely, and sensual muscles in about three to six months.

I have a sixty-one year old male client (*thin* body temple) who said, "I would like to see myself with a trim, healthy, fit body. I'm not trying to look like I'm thirty-five years old, but I want to look real good for sixty-one. I want to feel sexy when I take my shirt off. I want to look like you—just in the man version."

You probably have dreams of looking a certain way in less time than I recommend. Remember to work hard and consistently be patient. Your body will have more firm-shapely muscles, and less fat and cellulite before you know it. You'll look and feel younger and better.

Regaining a firm-body temple after few months of running and weight-training has been proven. Remember how I regained my firm-body temple after a year of no exercising. With retraining, it appears that my muscles remembered the work they did prior to the year off from training. Science must be correct about *muscle memory*—observation that weight-training muscles experience a rapid return of strength and muscle mass after lack of training for a while.

Did you notice I didn't say anything about the scale? That's because most bodybuilders, fitness and figure competitors, and athletes don't weigh themselves often. I check the mirror instead. I don't weigh myself often. What I view in mirrors and how my clothes fit are my measuring tools.

With patience, you'll be happy with what you view in your mirror, and how your clothes fit too.

I'M DETERMINED TO STAY FIT

Be somebody with a body. -Joe Weider
(Creator of Mr. Olympia and Ms. Olympia bodybuilding contests,
magazine publisher)

Don't be afraid...I am with you.
(Isaiah 43:1,4 and 44:2 NIV)

CHAPTER 10

FIRM-BODY TEMPLE WORKOUT

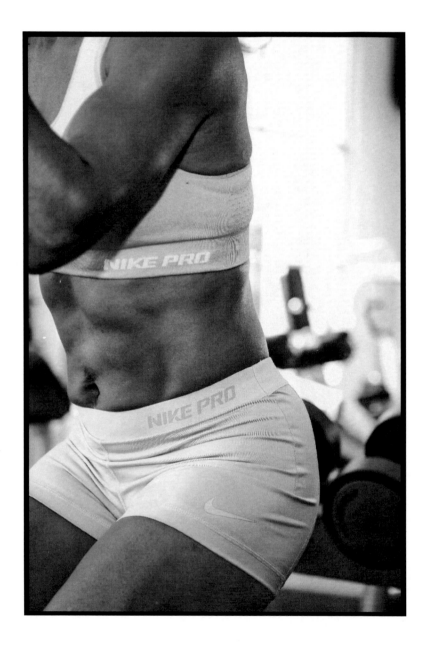

FIRST WEEK OF YOUR FIRM-BODY TEMPLE PROGRAM

Many people and I have transformed our body temples following revolutionary two and four days a week weight training programs. *Firm-Body Temple* is an innovative weight-training program that has been successfully tested with many people who saw amazing results in few months.

This program's designed just for you with couple options to save time and achieve similar/better results. You can work out two or four days per week. If you want to weight train two days per week, you'll workout your entire body temple by combining **Day 1 and Day 2 programs**, and completing both on the same day.

An hour and a half to two hours each day may be all you need to complete it. Note: The time depends on rest time between sets of exercises. You need to rest the next day (or the second) before doing the same routine again. You must allow your muscles to recuperate by resting at least a day or two after working out.

After resting for a day or two, complete the same Day 1 and 2 programs for one more day that week. For example, work out Monday, rest Tuesday, and work out again on Wednesday or Thursday. You can weight train all your muscle groups for a maximum of three days per week if you'd like, but you must rest the next day after your workout, if you want them to repair and grow.

If you prefer to train four days per week, complete the **Day 1 and Day 2 programs** on different days, twice per week. Joe Weider called this the *split routine*. This routine takes sixty to seventy-five minutes per workout. If you're in the gym, your total routine time may differ depending on how long you rest between sets, and wait for equipment. Perform Day 1 workout on Monday and Wednesday and Day 2 workout on Tuesday and Thursday. Rest on Friday and the weekend.

Note: Don't perform weight training on the same muscle groups two days in a row. Your abdominals are an exception. They can be exercised daily.

You'll break into your Firm-Body Temple-weight training program by performing only two sets for each exercise. This will allow you time to get well acquainted with your new workout routines, and start having fun working out with weights.

Although the Firm-Body Temple program was designed to use the *modified pyramiding* technique for each *set*, you may use the *pyramiding* technique. You'll do more work per set, as a result.

Pyramiding (also called stacking) is slightly increasing weights, and gradually decreasing the amount of weight until the initial weight is reached again, or a "*pyramid*" is achieved. *Pyramiding* is one of the best-kept secrets in the fitness industry. Many people in gyms are unfamiliar with it. Most athletes and bodybuilders use it to build and strengthen their body temples, and become champions.

Pyramiding is proven to be the most successful method to build, shape, and tone muscles successful because it plays mind games on your muscles. For instance, when your second set feels difficult, you tell yourself you can finish it because it's fewer reps than the first set. Then you'll work hard to finish it. You'll do the same for the final set. Although the weight is heavier, your muscles work to their maximum potential. With proper diet and *pyramiding*, the result is your firm-body temple.

This is an example of one *set* of leg extension with the *pyramiding* technique. First, extend the legs fifteen times with twenty pounds. Second, extend the legs ten times with twenty-five pounds. Third, extend the legs five times with thirty pounds. Fourth, extend the legs ten times with twenty-five pounds. Fifth, extend the legs fifteen times with twenty pounds. Rest five minutes. Repeat with two to three sets.

Pyramiding isn't useful for abdominals and buttocks exercises.

Modified pyramiding is helpful to remember what set you're working on because you're increasing the weight on the second and third sets.

Lift as follows: start with ten pounds if it's not heavy

Set 1: 12-15 reps with light weight (should feel easy - a natural warm up)

Set 2: 8-10 reps with heavier weights (increase weight 2.5, 5, or 10 pounds)

Set 3: 6-8 reps with heavier weights (increase weight 2.5, 5, or 10 pounds)

Note: If you're a beginning weight lifter, join my fitness classes, and/or book me for personal coaching (online or in person). I'll teach you how to perform the stretching, cardio, and weight training exercises in this book with ease. It's a practical investment for your health, safety, and wellbeing.

After your first week, perform three sets for each strength and weight training exercise. If you feel you're unready, don't perform three sets. On the other hand, at the start of your third week, start performing three sets for strength and weight-training exercises for optimal results.

You're starting with the leg exercises because they're bigger muscle groups, and may be more difficult to perform than your smaller ones. I prefer working on my legs first because they're more energized at the start of my workout. I enjoy my entire workout, as a result. You can start with any of the exercises in your program.

FIRM-BODY TEMPLE EXERCISE PROGRAM SUMMARY

It's essential to perform a minimum of two exercises per muscle group per day, twice per week to achieve firm, sexy, sensual muscles. Affirm yourself into shape by repeating affirmations before, during, and after your workouts.

DAY 1 (75-90 minutes)

LBBT Muscle Group (Legs, Buttocks, Biceps, Triceps)

LEGS

- Squat
- Leg Extensions (front upper legs)

LEGS, BUTTOCKS AND HIPS (Optional if Squats and Leg Extensions are sufficient)

- Lunges

- Rear Leg Extensions

CALVES

- Standing Toe Raises
- Seated Toe Raises

BICEPS

- Dumbbell Curls (Both arms or alternate arms)
- Concentration Curls (bench)

TRICEPS

- Dumbbell Kickbacks
- One Arm Dumbbell Extension

ABDOMINALS (ABS)

Perform two of the abs exercises (below) at the end of Day 1 and Day 2 workouts, if you're doing the four days per week program.

- Crunches (upper abs)
- Dumbbell Side Bends
- Seated Bent Knee Raises (lower abs)

Affirmation: I'm doing what it takes to firm my body.

FIRM-BODY TEMPLE EXERCISE PROGRAM SUMMARY

DAY 2 (60-75 minutes)

CBS Muscle Group (Chest, Back, Shoulders)

CHEST

- Dumbbell Press (Bench)
- Dumbbell Fly (Bench)

BACK

- One-Arm Dumbbell bent row (knee on bench)
- Bent Over Dumbbell Row (works abs, triceps, biceps, entire back)

SHOULDERS

- Alternate Dumbbell Raises (seated or standing) great for serratus/triceps too
- Dumbbell Side Lateral Raises

ABDOMINALS (ABS)

Perform two abs exercises (below). Perform on each workout day. No rest days are needed.

Disregard this entire "abs" section if you're using the two days a week program. You're performing abs on both of those workout days.

- Crunches (upper abs)
- Dumbbell Side Bends
- Seated Bent Knee Raises (lower abs)

Which one would you like to wear on your body temple?

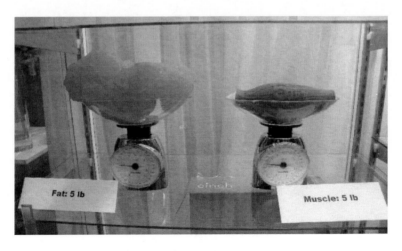

FAT VS MUSCLE (Anonymous source)

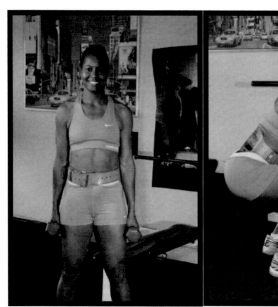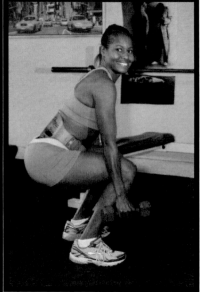

SQUAT

Affirmation: You can do it.

DAY 1 INSTRUCTIONS

SQUAT
QUADRICEPS, GLUTEUS MAXIMUS, HAMSTRINGS
EXERCISE 1

BUILDS, SHAPES, TONES: Quadriceps, Gluteus Maximus, and Hamstrings

PREPARE/POSITIONING: Stand in neutral position with your legs shoulder length apart. Hold the pair of dumbbells at your sides.

MOVEMENT: Keep your head upward. Slowly bend your knees. Lower your body until your legs are in ninety degree angle. Slowly raise back up to your starting position. Repeat.

CAUTION: Don't squat below your knees. You can injure them.

FOR VARIETY/EXTRAS: Use a block of wood under your heel for balance. Front Squat with dumbbells.

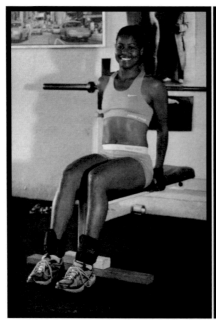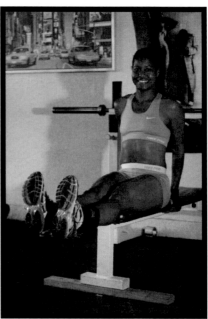

LEG EXTENSIONS

Affirmation: I'm determined to lose weight.

LEG EXTENSIONS
QUADRICEPS EXERCISE 2

BUILDS, SHAPES, TONES: Quadriceps

PREPARE/POSITIONING: Sit on a chair or bench with feet on the floor with the back of your knees against the seat. Strap on ankle weights. Keep back upright. Grasp the seat for balance.

MOVEMENT: Slowly raise your lower legs until both are fully contracted or parallel to the floor. Slowly return legs to the starting position. Repeat.

CAUTION: Don't lock your knees and raise lower legs fast. Don't drop legs to start position. Control the weight.

VARIETY/EXTRAS: Perform this exercise without weights. More repetitions burn more calories and tone muscles. Perform with one leg at a time.

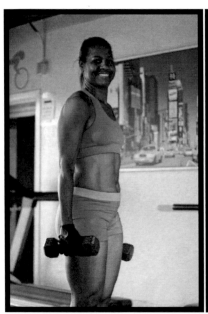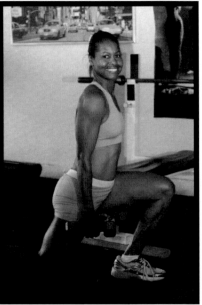

LUNGES

Affirmation: I'm doing what it takes to lose weight.

LUNGES
LEGS/BUTTOCKS/HIPS EXERCISE 1

BUILDS, SHAPES, TONES: Legs, buttocks, hips, abdominals

PREPARE/POSITIONING: Stand in neutral position with dumbbells in hands at your sides.

MOVEMENT: Slowly step forward with one leg, bent knee, and torso upright. Hold lead foot still with lead thigh parallel to the floor. Keep your rear leg stationary with knee almost touching the floor. Vigorously raise up to neutral position and repeat movement with other leg.

CAUTION: Don't step forward fast and never bounce. Don't bend your back when stepping forward. Keep your knees in line with your foot. Control movement with strength/coordination.

VARIETY/EXTRAS: Step on a (3-6 in. height) block of wood for a fuller stretch in your quadriceps muscles. Perform 3X12 reps with single leg. Use power cord with ankle cuffs to perform Side Leg Lifts. It's great for working your hips and outer thighs.

Affirmation: I feel great.

REAR LEG EXTENSIONS (with ankle weights)
LEGS/BUTTOCKS/HIPS EXERCISE 2

BUILDS, SHAPES, TONES: Legs, Buttocks, Hips

PREPARE/POSITIONING: Strap on ankle weights. Get down on both knees and hands on an exercise bench or exercise mat. Raise one leg into an *L* shape. Your raised thigh is parallel to the bench or floor.

MOVEMENT: Extend your leg upward, using your hip and buttock only. Straighten leg. Lift it high as possible. Remember to squeeze your buttocks while you lift. Return leg to start position. Repeat. Repeat movement with the alternate leg.

CAUTION: Movement may be uncomfortable at first, but don't quit. Don't let go of the *L* shape when at start position. Slowly and safely control the movement.

VARIETY/EXTRAS: Remember to complete this movement as described.

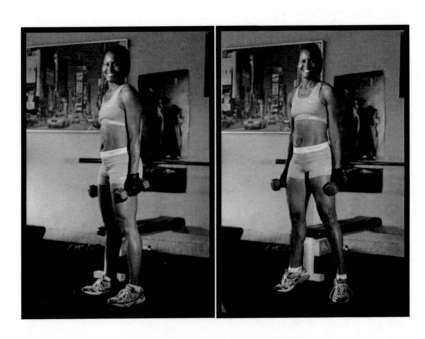

STANDING TOE RAISES

Affirmation: I'm determined to get firm.

STANDING TOE RAISES
CALVES EXERCISE 1

BUILDS, SHAPES, TONES: Calves

PREPARE/POSITIONING: Stand in neutral position on balls of feet on a block. Heels are on the floor. Grasp dumbbells at your sides.

MOVEMENT: Slowly raise your heels. Slowly lower your heels. Repeat.

CAUTION: Don't bounce or lock your knees.

VARIETY: Raise one heel at a time (alternate). Perform without wooden block. If you want large calves, lift heavier weights with fewer reps. If you want toned calves, lift lighter weights and perform more reps.

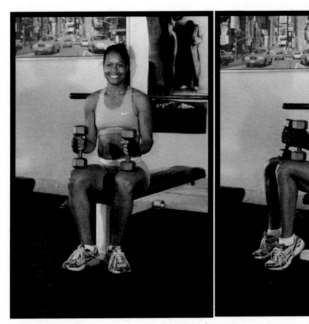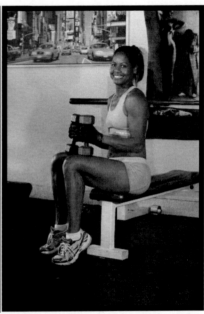

SEATED TOE RAISES

Affirmation: I'm powerful.

SEATED TOE RAISES
CALVES EXERCISE 2

BUILDS, SHAPES, TONES: Calves

PREPARE/POSITIONING: Sit on bench or chair with back upright. Grasp and place dumbbells on both thighs.

MOVEMENT: Slowly raise your heels. Slowly lower your heels. Repeat. Rest.

CAUTION: Don't use heavy dumbbells. They may bruise your thighs and be very uncomfortable. Don't bounce. Always grasp dumbbells during the movements.

VARIETY/EXTRAS: Alternate raising heels and hold for three seconds. Slowly lower heels. Repeat.

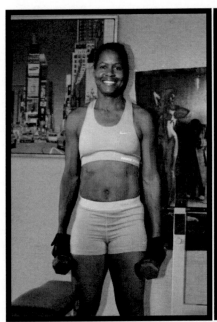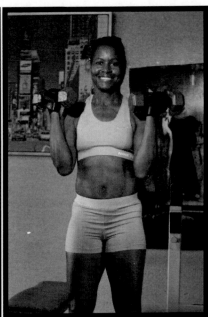

DUMBBELL CURLS

Affirmation: I'm spiritually strong.

DUMBBELL CURLS
BICEPS EXERCISE 1

BUILDS, SHAPES, TONES: Biceps

PREPARE/POSITIONING: Sit on a chair or edge of a bench holding dumbbells with hands turned outward. Start with straight arms near your sides and dumbbells in each hand. You can stand while holding the dumbbells. Beginners can use a couple tomato paste cans as weights. Back is upright, inner arms are pinned to your sides, and elbows bent. Perform in front of a mirror.

MOVEMENT: Slowly raise (curl) lower arms to shoulders. Squeeze (flex) biceps. Slowly lower dumbbells to start position. Repeat. Let the dumbbell stretch biceps on the return position.

CAUTION: Always control the dumbbells. Keep inner arms pinned to sides during the exercise. Never lock elbows or drop the dumbbells on the return to start the position. Don't push elbows outward when curling dumbbells.

VARIETY/EXTRAS: Perform Alternating Dumbbell Curls standing with legs shoulder width apart. For more challenge, pause (2-3 seconds) and squeeze biceps when dumbbells are near shoulders. Use a power cord too.

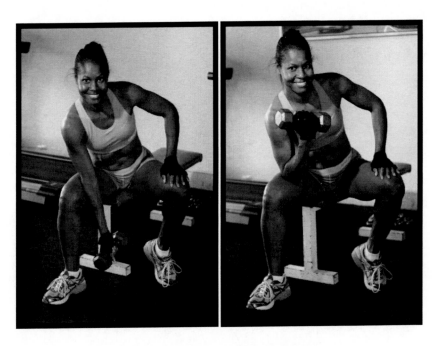

CONCENTRATION CURLS

Affirmation: I'm determined to become sexy.

CONCENTRATION CURLS
BICEPS EXERCISE 2

BUILDS, SHAPES, TONES: Biceps

PREPARE/POSITIONING: Sit on a bench or chair. Hold a dumbbell in right hand. Extend right arm forward with palm up. Sit with legs slightly apart. Position left hand on left thigh.

MOVEMENT: Slowly raise right arm (curl) near right shoulder. Remember to squeeze bicep. Slowly return it to start position. Repeat. Switch and repeat with left arm.

CAUTION: Always control dumbbell. Don't jerk or swing dumbbell or drop it on the return.

VARIETY: Perform exercise standing up and slightly leaning forward. Perform Barbell Curls with a barbell. Then stand and curl with both hands.

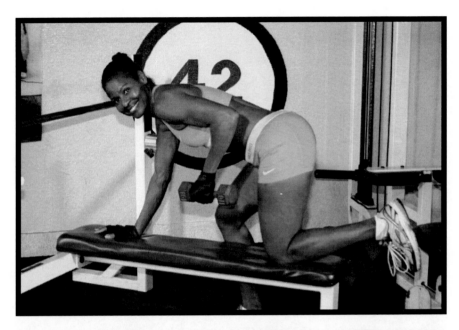

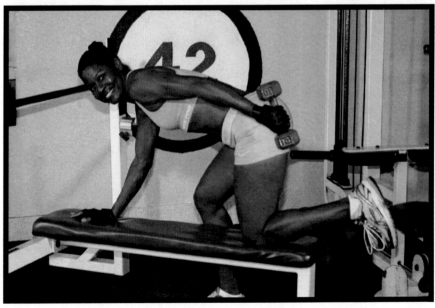

DUMBBELL KICKBACKS

DUMBBELL KICKBACKS (BENCH)
TRICEPS EXERCISE 1

BUILDS, SHAPES, TONES: Triceps

PREPARE/POSITIONING: Kneel with left knee on bench. Left hand is flat on bench. Hold a dumbbell in right hand with bent elbow. Right knee has slight bend. Back is parallel to the bench.

MOVEMENT: Keep elbow close to your waist. Slowly extend dumbbell straight back. Slowly return it to start position. Repeat. Switch to left arm. Repeat movement.

CAUTION: Always control dumbbell. Don't swing dumbbell or lock elbows. Correct form is essential for your safety.

VARIETY: Perform exercise without a bench. Use power cord to perform Triceps Kickbacks.

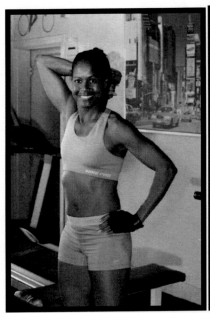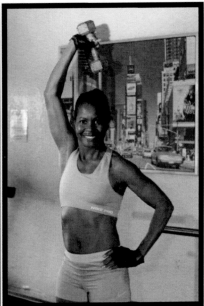

ONE-ARM DUMBBELL EXTENSION

Affirmation: I am what I am.

ONE-ARM DUMBBELL EXTENSION
TRICEPS EXERCISE 2

BUILDS, SHAPES, TONES: Triceps

PREPARE/POSITIONING: Stand in front of a mirror in neutral position, or be seated. Hold one dumbbell with straight arm above your head. Keep triceps very close to ear. Palm faces the mirror. Chest is upright. Your free hand on your closest or opposite hip.

MOVEMENT: Slowly bend your elbow. Carefully lower the weight behind your head. Slowly extend your arm with dumbbell to start position. Squeeze your triceps. Repeat. Switch to the other arm after finishing that set.

CAUTION: Don't drop the weight when you lower it. Don't lock your elbows.

VARIETY: Perform Seated Dumbbell Extension with both hands. (See Bonus Exercises for Troubled Body Parts) Use a barbell to perform same movement with both hands. Use power cord to perform One-Arm Extension.

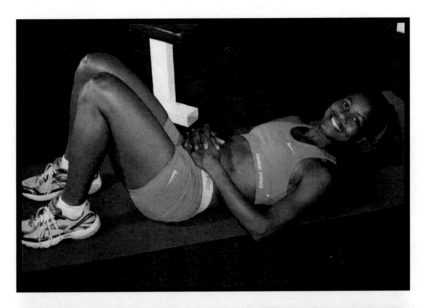

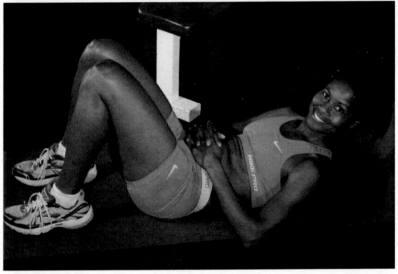

CRUNCHES

Affirmation: I'm transforming my abs.

CRUNCHES (OR RAISED LEGS CRUNCHES)
ABDOMINALS EXERCISE 1

BUILDS, SHAPES, TONES: Abdominals

NOTE: With low calorie/fat diet and cardio exercises, crunches are more effective to build fit, "six pack" or "washboard" abs. They engage abs more than planks.

PREPARE/POSITIONING: Lie with head and back on floor and bent knees, and/or calves resting on a bench or standard-size chair. Arms at your sides, or hands on your lower abdominals. Hands may be connected behind your head for balance.

MOVEMENT: Slowly curl upper torso until shoulder blades are off floor. Slowly return shoulder blades to the floor. Feel the *pump*. Focus on only your abs doing the work. Repeat. Try to complete 25 repetitions per set, without resting. As your abs get stronger, complete 50 reps per set.

CAUTION: Don't raise your back off the floor. Don't use hands and arms to pull torso off floor. Don't thrust off the floor. If neck is uncomfortable, support it with your hands.

VARIETY: Perform exercise with knees up or legs straight up to sky. This exercise will build upper and lower abs.

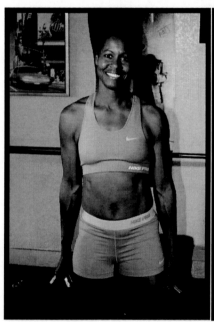 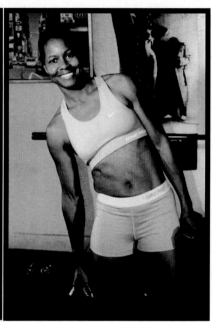

DUMBBELL SIDE BEND
(START POSITION)

DUMBBELL SIDE BEND
(END POSITION)

Affirmation: I've got this!

DUMBBELL SIDE BEND
ABDOMINALS EXERCISE 2

BUILDS, SHAPES, TONES: Abdominals

PREPARE/POSITIONING: Stand upright holding a dumbbell in each hand extended at your side with legs shoulder width apart.

MOVEMENT: Slowly bend your torso to your right side. Then to the left side. Keep your arms extended by your side. Allow the weights to pull you downward. Repeat by alternating sides. Rest.

CAUTION: Always control the weight. Never jerk the weight.

VARIETY: Perform the exercise on your right side for a full set. Then switch to your left side for a full set.

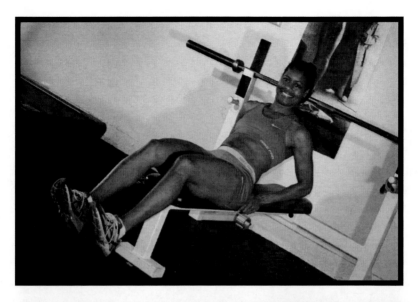

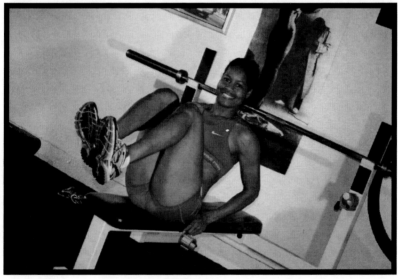

SEATED BENT KNEE RAISES (KNEE UPS)

Affirmation: I'm shattering fat!

SEATED BENT KNEE RAISES (KNEE UPS)
ABDOMINALS EXERCISE 3

BUILDS, SHAPES, TONES: Lower Abdominals, hips, adductors

PREPARE/POSITIONING: Sit on bench with knees slightly bent and lower legs extended in front of you. Position hands on sides of bench, right behind buttocks. Lean backwards.

MOVEMENT: Slowly raise knees toward chest. Slowly return legs to start position. Repeat. Try to complete 25 repetitions per set to start. As your abs get stronger, complete 50 reps per set.

CAUTION: Always control movements. Grasp bench firmly for balance and support. Don't rush the movement. Don't drop feet to the floor during the exercise--except for pain..

VARIETY: Perform exercise with ankle cuff weights for more challenge. Raise legs to hips and crunch torso.

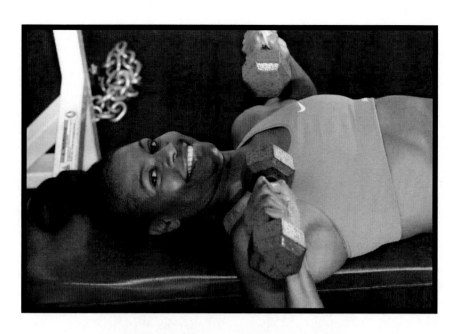

DUMBBELL PRESS (START POSITION)

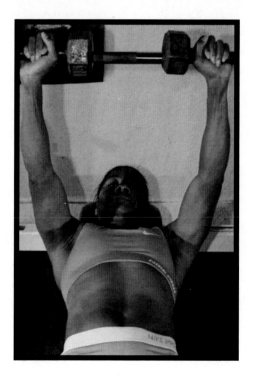

DUMBBELL PRESS (END POSITION)

CBS (Chest, Back, Shoulders Exercise Routine)

Perform CBS on different days than LBBT (Legs, Buttocks, Biceps, Triceps) Routines
(Two times per week)

DUMBBELL PRESS
CHEST EXERCISE 1

BUILDS, SHAPES, TONES: Chest, Triceps minimally, Serratus minimally.

PREPARE POSITIONING: Lie on the bench holding dumbbells above chest. Knees are bent, and feet are flat on floor.

MOVEMENT: Slowly bend arms. Lower the dumbbells close to chest. Slowly push dumbbells back to start position. Repeat.

CAUTION: Control the dumbbells. Always use a spotter (person to assist) when lifting heavy weights. Don't lower the dumbbells quickly. Don't let your elbows drop below your body. Think about your chest doing the work.

VARIETY: Use a barbell with plates on both sides.

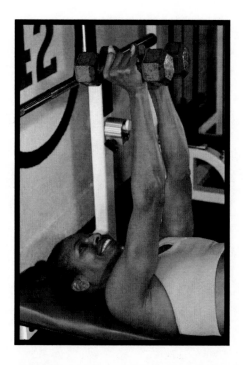

DUMBBELL FLY (START POSITION)

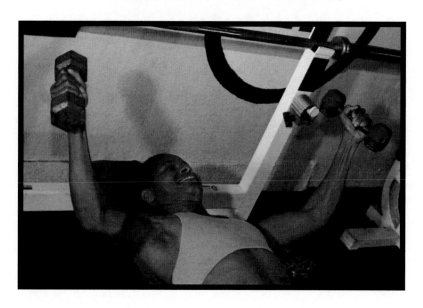

DUMBBELL FLY (END POSITION)

Affirmation: I'm determined to have a firm body!

DUMBBELL FLY (BENCH)
CHEST EXERCISE 2

BUILDS, SHAPES, TONES: Chest, Triceps, Serratus

PREPARE/POSITIONING: Lie with your back arched on a bench. Hold two dumbbells above chest. Slightly bend elbows.

MOVEMENT: Slowly lower the dumbbells outward (arclike position). Keep dumbbells at above chest. Slowly press the dumbbells up to the start position. Repeat.

CAUTION: Control the dumbbells with every movement. Never lower them quickly.

VARIETY: Use an incline bench. Use power cord to perform Fly.

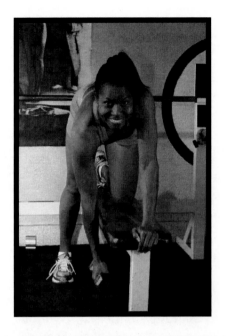

ONE-ARM DUMBBELL ROW (START)

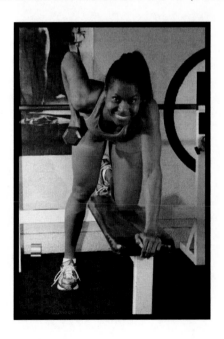

ONE-ARM DUMBBELL ROW (END POSITION)

Affirmation: I'm sexy!

ONE-ARM DUMBBELL ROW
LATISSIMUS DORSI EXERCISE 1

BUILDS, SHAPES, TONES: Latissimus dorsi (Lats give the core *V*-shape look)

PREPARE/POSITIONING: Hold a dumbbell downward with a straight right arm. Kneel with left knee on bench and right leg straight. Left hand is positioned flat on bench. Right foot is flat on the floor.

MOVEMENT: Slowly pull the dumbbell to your waist with elbows bent. Slowly return dumbbell to the start position. Let it pull your arm straight down and stretch your back. Switch to the left hand. Repeat movements.

CAUTION: Always control the dumbbell. Don't let it drop when returning to the start position. Keep your back and head parallel to the bench.

VARIETY: Perform same movement (while standing) in a slightly bent position with dumbbells in each hand. Pull and lower the dumbbells to and from your waist. Use power cord.

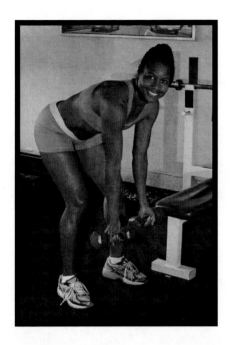

BENT OVER ROW (START POSITION)

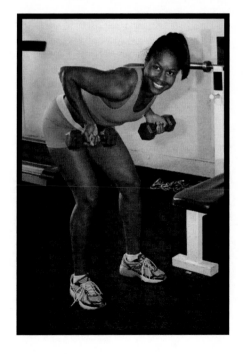

BENT OVER ROW (END POSITION)

Affirmation: I'm powerful!

BENT OVER ROW
LATISSIMUS DORSI EXERCISE 2

BUILDS, SHAPES, TONES: Latissimus, Biceps, Deltoids, Abdominals

PREPARE/POSITIONING: Hold dumbbells with arms to sides. Stand with legs shoulder-width apart and knees slightly bent. Keep back slightly bent and head up.

MOVEMENT: Lean forward. Slowly pull both dumbbells near ribcage. Slowly return dumbbells to the start position.

CAUTION: Always control the dumbbells. Don't drop dumbbells to starting position. Keep back straight when bent over. Keep knees slightly bent during exercise.

VARIETY: Use barbell to perform exercise and have more control. Use a power cord to perform.

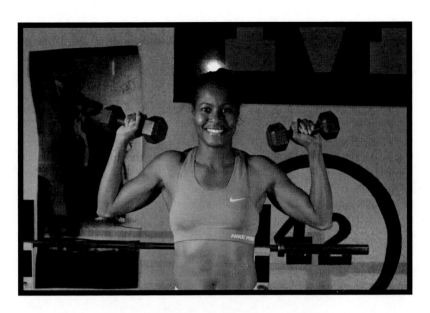

ALTERNATE DUMBBELL PRESS (START POSITION)

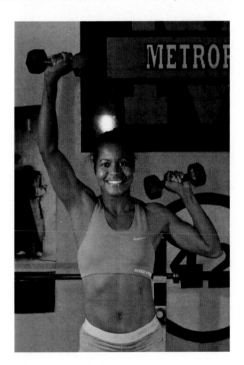

ALTERNATE DUMBBELL PRESS (END POSITION)

Affirmation: I'm sexy!

ALTERNATE DUMBBELL PRESS
(Great three-in-one exercise!)
DELTOIDS EXERCISE 1

BUILDS, SHAPES, TONES: Deltoids, triceps, and serratus

PREPARE/POSITIONING: Sit upright on a bench or chair holding the dumbbells above your shoulders or about ear level. You can stand too. Feet are flat on the floor.

MOVEMENT: Start with the dumbbells slightly above your shoulders. Slowly PRESS the right dumbbell straight up while you hold the left or alternate dumbbell at about ear level. Slowly return the dumbbell to the start position. Alternate with the left dumbbell with same movement until your set is complete.

CAUTION: Control the dumbbells. Never rush your movements. Don't lock your elbows. Sit upright looking straight ahead.

VARIETY: Perform movement standing with legs shoulder width apart.

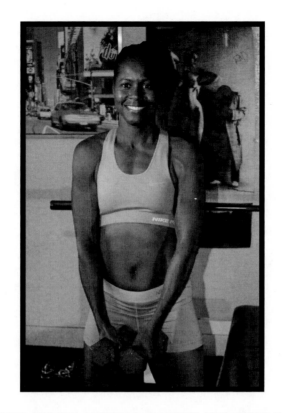

DUMBBELL SIDE LATERAL RAISES (START POSITION)

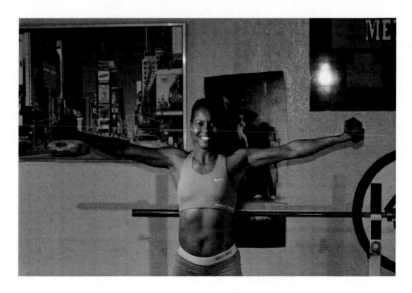

DUMBBELL SIDE LATERAL RAISES (END POSITION)

Affirmation: I'm fit and fabulous!

DUMBBELL SIDE LATERAL RAISES
DELTOIDS EXERCISE 2

BUILDS, SHAPES, TONES: Deltoids, trapezius

PREPARE/POSITIONING: Stand with legs shoulder width apart. Hold dumbbells in front of thighs. Lean forward slightly. Bend knees slightly.

MOVEMENT: Slowly RAISE the dumbbells laterally (outward and upward) to shoulder level. Palms are facing floor. Keep your elbows slightly bent. Slowly return them to starting position. Flex your shoulders on the upward movement. Stretch your shoulders on the downward movement. Repeat.

CAUTION: Always control dumbbells with slow movements. If pyramiding, start with light weight. If heavy, it's difficult to get a full raise. Don't lock your elbows or swing arms. Keep your knees slightly bent.

VARIETY: Perform while seated on bench or chair. Perform movement with one arm at a time for one set. Then repeat with the alternate arm. Use dumbbells or power cord to perform. Alternate Front Raise or Front Raise (both hands) by raising dumbbell in front of or away from you.

Affirmation: I've got this!

NOTE: Perform 2 of the 3 abs exercises below. No rest is needed on each workout day because these are small muscles. **See DAY 1 INSTRUCTIONS and images for abs workout directions (in this chapter).**

CRUNCHES (OR RAISED LEGS CRUNCHES)
ABDOMINALS EXERCISE 1

DUMBBELL SIDE BEND
ABDOMINALS EXERCISE 2

SEATED BENT KNEE RAISES (KNEE UPS)
ABDOMINALS EXERCISE 3

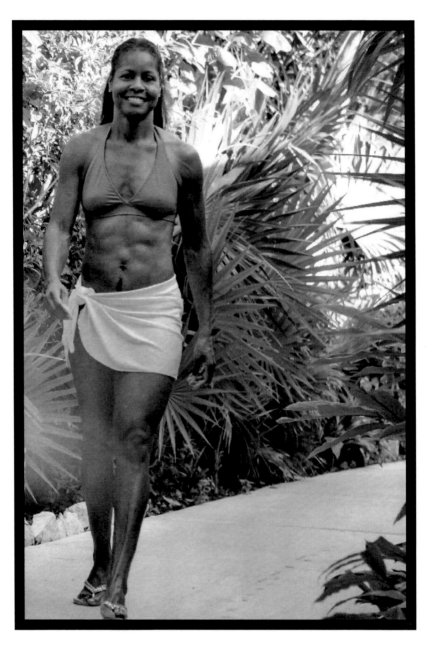

The fat of his body will waste away.
(Isaiah 17:4 NIV Bible)

I'M HAPPY WITH MY FIT ABS!

CHAPTER 11

BONUS EXERCISES FOR TROUBLED PARTS

If you're like me, you're probably eager to see quick results in those displeasing parts of your body temple. To reach your goal, you will need to perform additional exercises and extend your workout time.

This chapter provides the additional exercises necessary to achieve faster results. You can add them to your regular routine from the previous chapter. Perform them on the same day that you're working on that body part.

For instance, if you want to see faster results on your triceps, add Seated Dumbbell Extension and/or Push Ups from this chapter to your Kickbacks and Dips. Perform a minimum of three to four exercises per muscle group to get maximum results.

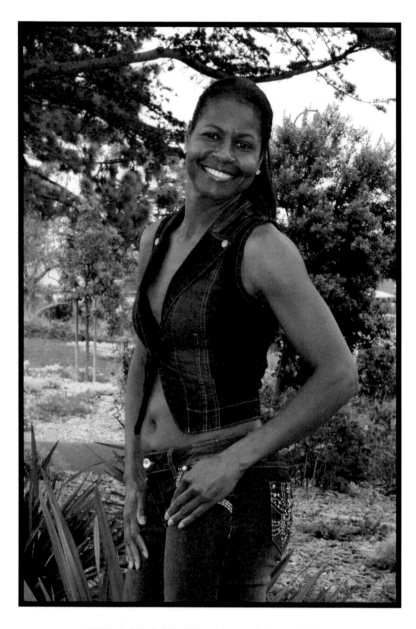

AFFIRM YOURSELF INTO SHAPE. ™

TROUBLED PARTS EXERCISE PROGRAM SUMMARY

TRICEPS AND BICEPS

Push-Ups (Four-in-One Exercise for chest, back, front, and rear arms)
Seated Dumbbell Extensions (Both hands holding a dumbbell behind head)
Dips (With bent knees)

GLUTEUS MAXIMUS, HIPS, HAMSTRINGS

Belize Buttocks Squeeze TM (BBS)
Rear Leg Extension

HAMSTRINGS AND GLUTEUS MAXIMUS

Leg Curl
Wide-Leg Dumbbell Squat

ABDOMINALS

Cross Over Crunches
Standing Leg Lifts
Planks

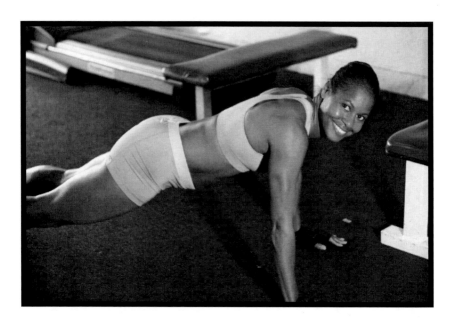

PUSH-UPS (START POSITION)

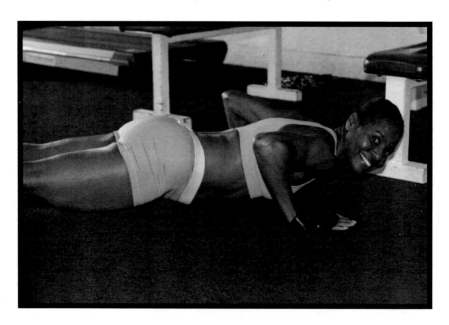

PUSH-UPS (END POSITION)

Affirmation: I'm determined to be fit!

PUSH-UPS
CHEST, SHOULDERS, BICEPS, TRICEPS EXERCISE 1
(Four-in-One Exercise)

BUILDS, SHAPES, TONES: Chest, Shoulders, Biceps, Triceps

PREPARE/POSITIONING: Place knees and hands on floor or exercise mat and feet against a wall. Your legs, abdominals, and chest are raised—almost parallel to the floor.

MOVEMENT: Slowly bend your elbows and lower your body close to the floor or exercise mat. Push up your body with your arms to start position. Keep your feet positioned on the wall until each set is completed. Your body barely touches the floor or exercise mat.

CAUTION: Don't let your chest, abdominals, and knees touch to the floor. Always control your body. Don't do push-ups with your knees on the floor or what some call Girl Push-Ups. Get faster results.

VARIETY: If this is your first time performing push-ups, do as many as you can. Your arms will get stronger.

In a 2012 push-up contest, then First Lady Michelle Obama, executed twenty-five push-ups (or press-ups) nonstop on *The Ellen Degeneres Show*. Ellen executed twenty. Ellen joked, "I thought it wouldn't be good to show up the First Lady, so I stopped. I thought this looks bad that I'm going to beat her." (Time Magazine)

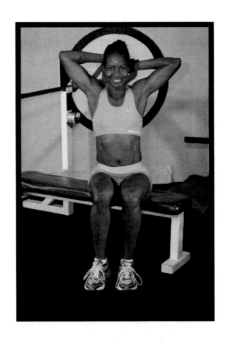

SEATED DUMBBELL EXTENSION
START POSITION

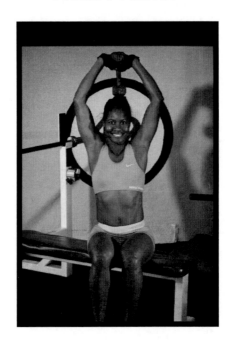

END POSITION

Affirmation: I'm determined to get stronger!

SEATED DUMBBELL EXTENSION
TRICEPS EXERCISE 2

BUILDS, SHAPES, TONES: Triceps

PREPARE/POSITIONING: Sit on a bench or chair with both arms extended over your head. Hold a dumbbell behind your head with both hands.

MOVEMENT: Slowly lower your forearms with dumbbell behind you. Slowly extend dumbbell to start position. Repeat. Rest.

CAUTION: Always control the weight. Never let the weight drop behind you to prevent injury.

VARIETY: Perform exercise standing upright with feet in neutral position. Use power cord to perform One-Arm Extensions.

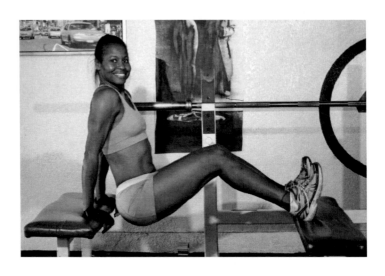

DIPS (START POSITION)

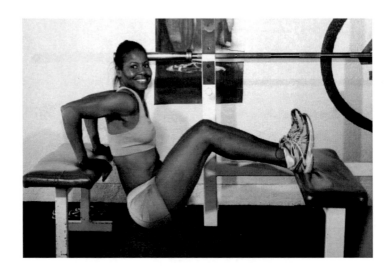

DIPS (END POSITION)

Affirmation: I'm determined to be healthier!

DIPS (WITH BENT KNEES)

IMPORTANT: If you don't have two benches, use two stable chairs to hold your bodyweight.

TRICEPS EXERCISE 2

BUILDS, SHAPES, TONES: Triceps

PREPARE/POSITIONING: Place palm of hands on edge of a chair. Arms are straight. Head and chest are upright. Place heels on top of the other chair. Knees are slightly bent.

MOVEMENT: Slowly bend elbows and lower body until upper arms are parallel to floor. Slowly push back up and straighten arms. Don't lock your elbows when you return to the start position. Repeat.

CAUTION: Always control the movements. Never jerk up to the start position. Don't lower your body too fast. You may injure your shoulders and elbows. This movement may be difficult in the beginning.

VARIETY: Move your grasp to different positions on the chair. Position a dumbbell on your lap to challenge yourself. Use the Pyramiding technique with dumbbell in your lap. Perform Triceps Kickbacks with power cords.

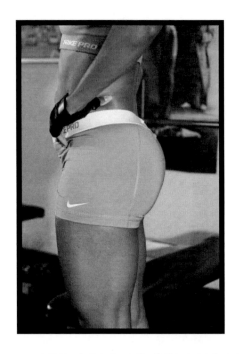

BELIZEAN BUTT SQUEEZE (START POSITION)

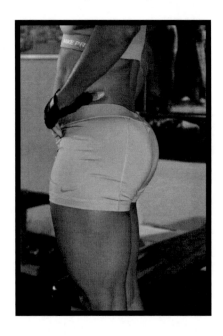

BELIZEAN BUTT SQUEEZE OR BBS (END POSITION)

Affirmation: I'm determined to have a firm butt!

BELIZEAN BUTT SQUEEZE (BBS)TM
BUTTOCKS/LEGS/HIPS EXERCISE 1

BUILDS, SHAPES, TONES: Buttocks, Hips, Legs

PREPARE/POSITIONING: Stand with the legs in neutral position. Slightly bend your knees. Arms are at your sides.

MOVEMENT: Squeeze buttocks tightly for about two seconds. Relax. Repeat until the set is complete.

CAUTION: Don't raise your heels when squeezing your buttocks. Visualize your buttocks looking tight and round like an onion, or basketball.

VARIETY: Place your hands on your hips and squeeze your buttocks tightly. Behave like you're posing in your swimsuit photo shoot. Have fun! Use power cord with ankle cuffs to perform Glute Kickbacks while standing behind and holding a chair, or hands are on a wall.

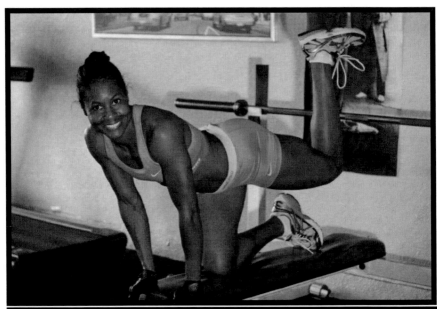

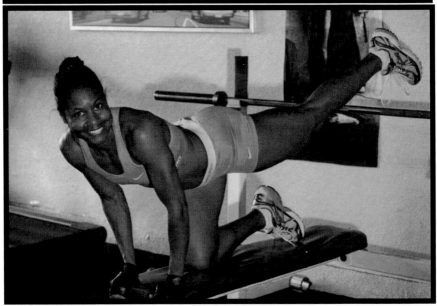

REAR LEG EXTENSION
(START POSITION AT THE TOP. END POSITION IS ABOVE)

Affirmation: My body temple is firm!

REAR LEG EXTENSION (with or without ankle weights)
BUTTOCKS/LEGS/HIPS EXERCISE 2

BUILDS, SHAPES, TONES: Buttocks, Hips, Legs

PREPARE/POSITIONING: Strap on ankle weights. Get down on both knees and hands on an exercise bench or mat. Raise one leg into an *L* shape. Your raised thigh is parallel to the bench or floor.

MOVEMENT: Extend your leg upward, using your hip and buttock only. Straighten leg. Lift it high as possible. Remember to squeeze your buttocks while you lift. Return leg to start position. Repeat. Then repeat movement with the alternate leg.

CAUTION: Don't let go of the L shape when at start position. Slowly and safely control the movement.

VARIETY/EXTRAS: Use power cord with ankle cuffs to perform Glute Kickbacks while standing behind and holding a chair or hands are on a wall.

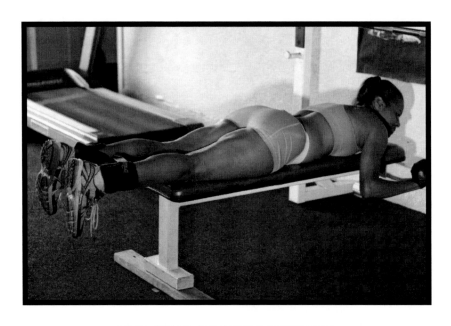

LEG CURL (START POSITION)

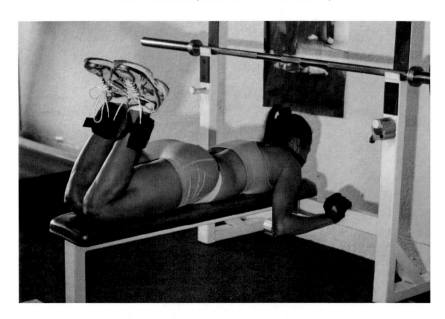

LEG CURL (END POSITION)

Affirmation: I'm determined to have firm legs!

LEG CURL (WITH ANKLE WEIGHTS)
HAMSTRINGS EXERCISE 1

BUILDS, SHAPES, TONES: Hamstrings

PREPARE/POSITIONING: Strap on ankle cuff weights. Lie, facedown, on a padded exercise bench, with knees and legs off the bench. Extend legs parallel to the floor. Grip the front of the bench with your hands.

MOVEMENT: Slowly bend your knees and raise your heels to your buttocks. Slowly lower your lower legs to the start position. Repeat.

CAUTION: Always control the weight. Never rush the movements of the weights or drop your legs quickly to start position.

VARIETY: Perform this exercise without weights and do as many repetitions as possible. Rest. Repeat. Have a partner hold your lower leg. Slowly bend your knees and raise your heels to your buttocks. Repeat.

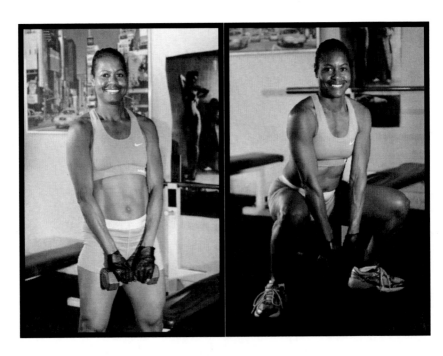

DUMBBELL WIDE-LEG SQUAT
[START AND END POSITION (ON RIGHT)]

Affirmation: I'm determined to have sexy legs and butt!

DUMBBELL WIDE-LEG SQUAT
QUADRICEPS, ADDUCTORS, BUTTOCKS, AND
HAMSTRINGS EXERCISE 2

BUILDS, SHAPES, TONES: Quadriceps, Adductors, Buttocks, Hamstrings, and Abdominals

PREPARE/POSITIONING: Stand with legs slightly more than shoulder width apart with toes pointed outward. Hold a dumbbell in front of you with both hands.

MOVEMENT: Slowly bend your knees and lower your body until your thighs are parallel to the floor or are in an *L* position. Imagine that you're sitting on a chair. Keep your chest and back as upright as possible. Slowly stand up and return to start position. Feel your inner thighs working and tightening. Repeat. Rest. Use power cord with ankle cuffs too. They're great for working your hips and outer thighs.

CAUTION: Don't spread your legs too wide (prevents knee injury). Always control the weight. Never stand up quickly or lock knees.

VARIETY: Do Super Burn sets by performing this exercise without weight until your leg and buttocks feel like they're burning. Rest for 30 seconds.

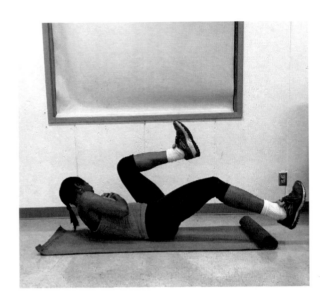

CROSSOVER CRUNCHES

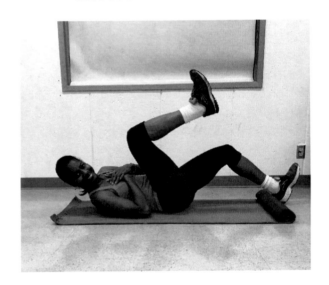

CROSSOVER CRUNCHES

Affirmation: I'm determined to have firm abs!

CROSSOVER CRUNCHES
ABDOMINALS EXERCISE 1

BUILDS, SHAPES, TONES: Abdominals

PREPARE/POSITIONING: Lie on your back with your feet flat on exercise mat. Place hands on chest or behind head. Keep your arms and elbows extended—parallel to the mat.

MOVEMENT: Slowly raise your right shoulder. Cross over to your left side. Slowly lower your right shoulder to the mat. Switch to your left shoulder. Cross over to your right side. Slowly return left shoulder to the mat. Complete set. Repeat. Rest.

CAUTION: Don't raise your back off the mat.

VARIETY: Extend right leg and bring left knee toward your core, or trunk. Alternate legs while crossing over. When you extend legs, keep feet about six inches off floor. Use a power cord to perform Standing Twist.

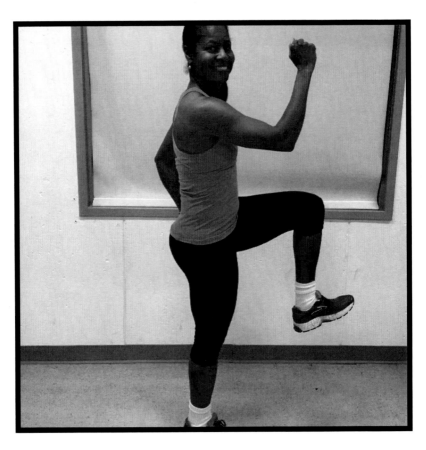

STANDING LEG LIFT

Affirmation: I feel great!

STANDING LEG LIFT (KNEE RAISES)
ABDOMINALS EXERCISE 2

BUILDS, SHAPES, TONES: Abdominals

PREPARE/POSITIONING: Stand with legs shoulder. Arms extended to your sides for balance.

MOVEMENT: Slowly raise right knee to hip. Lower right leg to the floor. Slowly raise left knee to hip. Lower left leg to the floor. Rest. Repeat.

CAUTION: Don't drop leg quickly to the floor.

VARIETY: Perform exercise with ankle cuff weights for more challenge. Stand in a doorway to perform this exercise. Hold onto the doorjamb if support is necessary.

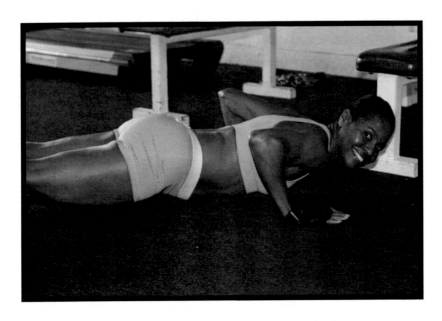

PLANK (HOLD THIS POSITION)

Affirmation: I'm determined to have sexy abs!

PLANK (PUSH-UP POSITION)
ABDOMINALS EXERCISE 3

BUILDS, SHAPES, TONES: Abdominals and obliques

Note: Crunches are more effective than planks to build "six pack," "washboard," and flat abs. They engage abs more than planks would. Planks are effective for strengthening and toning abs.

PREPARE/POSITIONING: A stop watch is needed for timing. Get into push-up position on floor. Your hips are tucked under and spine's straight.

MOVEMENT: Hold body up on both forearms and toes. Remain still. Keep spine straight. Hold position for 30 or more seconds. When done, go down to start position. Rest for couple minutes. Repeat two more sets.

CAUTION: Don't arch your spine or raise buttocks. If your body's trembling, control it as best you can.

VARIETY: Hold plank position and turn to right side. Lift one arm upward to the sky. Balance on one forearm. Hold your body straight, without arching or sagging your trunk or core. Hold as long as you can. Switch to the left side. Slowly lower your body down. Rest.

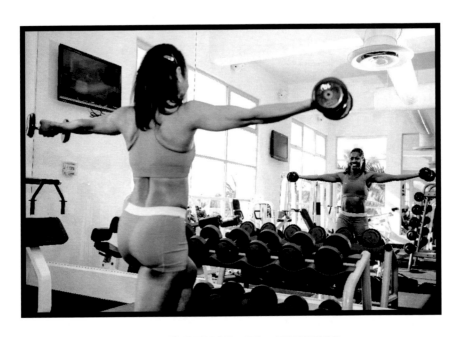

80% NUTRITION + 20% FITNESS = BODY TEMPLE APPEARANCE

When I choose healthy foods and water, I'm the best doctor and nutritionist for me. -Althea Moses

CHAPTER 12

NUTRITIONAL CHOICES

This isn't a comprehensive nutritional food choices chapter. It started out that way. I wrote seventy-five detailed pages about nutrition for men and women. Then I realized that all of the information written was unnecessary for a book about building the spirit and physical body temple with exercises. I condensed it to teach you some of the most important things you need to become irresistibly fit forever. See my next book on nutrition.

This chapter includes: importance and functions of calories, three sources of calorie burning that's influenced by your muscle mass, how to lose weight with the Hamwi Equation, and three important nutrients.

Making healthy food and water choices are essential to achieving your firm-body temple building goals. When shopping for food and water, ask yourself, "Why do I put quality gas and oil in my car and not quality foods and water in my body temple?

Your body temple needs a balance of nutrition to lose excess fat and maintain your health. Your physical activities and recovery are enhanced by optimal nutrition. I recommend appropriate selection of food and water and supplement choices for optimal health and exercise performance.

Often, many of my clients stated that their lifestyles are so busy there isn't enough time to prepare and eat great tasting, healthy foods. So I asked, "Is that what you were going for? Are you happy with that?" Their answer is always, "No." Then, I educate them about calorie functions and the importance of choosing nutritional foods and water.

CALORIES

Calorie balance is one of the most important aspect of your healthy-nutritional choices. Every body temple needs energy or calories to function properly and what is more important, to stay alive. Calories are units of energy your body temple takes and burns for energy—from your consumed food and beverages. NOTE: All calories aren't equal, so choose wisely.

If you want to live a moderate to high quality of life, you need to know and do what it takes to acquire your daily requirement of calories. Since body temple compositions are different, everyone needs different amounts of calories to function. In fact, you need calories to sustain your body functions as you rest (while awake) and literally sleeping. Research shows about forty calories per hour are burned while we sleep. If you're weight training, you burn even more calories per hour—about sixty calories.

More specifically, our bodies need calories for involuntary functions like: breathing, digestion of foods and water, maintenance of heart rate, blood pressure and body temperature. That's the reason many people (in hospitals), who are unable to eat foods are fed intravenously. Calories aren't our enemy. They're our best friends. We need them to survive.

On the other hand, consuming too many calories can be harmful to your body temple. It responds by storing excess calories as fat (in fat cells) as a way to protect itself from a future famine. "You're programmed to put on fat whenever there's food available, but now there's a lot of food available, but it's the wrong kind," according to Dr. Christiane Northrup, New York Times best-selling author of *Women's Bodies, Women's Wisdom*.

Your goal is to reduce excess calories, consume nutrient-rich calories and water, and build functional lean muscle mass to lose weight and the soft unattractive fat on your body temple. You can't spot reduce any part of your body. It doesn't work.

KEY: You'll need to burn 3,500 excess calories to lose one pound of body fat. For example, if you have excess of one pound of body fat, you'll need to burn about 500 excess calories per day to lose it in about a week. You can achieve that and much more with cardio and weight training.

Cardiovascular activities will burn calories while you're exercising. Weight or strength training will burn calories during exercise and while you're relaxing on your sofa and asleep on your bed. According to the American College of Sports Medicine (ACSM), functional lean muscle mass burns more calories than fat. Furthermore, muscles burn calories, whereas fat just stores them. Muscles hold more water.

Perform strength, weight or resistance training exercises to burn more calories, lose more weight, build functional-lean muscle mass, and remain hydrated, so that you can have a firm-body temple and all of the health benefits.

THREE EFFECTIVE WAYS TO MANAGE YOUR WEIGHT FOREVER

1. BASAL METABOLIC RATE FUNCTION (BMR)

BMR is the amount of energy your body temple expends (uses up) and needs at rest (awake or asleep) to stay alive. Don't be alarmed because this nutritional program does not expect you to count calories often. However, you should know how calories work and how much you need to prevent your body temple from getting excess fat—to remain irresistibly fit, healthy, and strong forever.

Your daily caloric need is determined by your basal metabolic rate (BMR), age, gender, functional lean muscle mass, exercise, and voluntary movement (also called NEAT or Non Exercise Activity Thermogenesis). Couple examples of NEAT are fidgeting and pacing.

There are three sources of calorie burning influenced by your muscle mass: basal metabolic rate (BMR), thermic effect of food, and physical activity or exercise. All of your involuntary functions affect your BMR.

Your body burns calories from your consumed foods (comprised of carbohydrates, fat, and protein). BMR is responsible (in most of us) for about sixty to seventy-five percent of our daily energy expenditure needs, so it's critical. Since it is, you should consume nutritionally high calorie foods and beverages--and avoid foods and sweetened beverages with empty calories.

What determines your BMR? Your muscle mass determines your BMR. It's a very critical part of burning calories and building and maintaining your firm-body temple.

For many people it's challenging to determine the amount of calories needed to consume and expend. Use this book to make it easier and get the results you need.

You'll put together your own pack of total energy intake and expenditure and make it work for you. Your total energy intake is determined by the number of calories you consume. Your total expenditure of calories is determined by your BMR, thermic effect of food, and physical activity level. Start by calculating your BMR to get better results today.

How do you determine your necessary BMR calories? Use this method, **Hamwi Equation** (for adults), to determine your (estimated) daily amount of calories needed for your BMR and Ideal Body Weight. Use your height to start. First, women should write 100 pounds for the first five feet of height and add five pounds for each inch after five feet of height.

For example, my height is about five feet eight inches. I'll write 100 pounds for my first five feet of height. Then multiply eight inches times five pounds, which is forty pounds. Finally I'll add 100 pounds and forty pounds together. This makes my "ideal body weight" 140 pounds. My "exact or actual weight" is 150 pounds, but it's unnecessary for this equation. Then I'll multiply 140 times ten. This is 1,400. This is my BMR or amount of calories I need at rest and to stay alive daily. Knowing this number helps me to make better nutritional choices and remain irresistibly fit.

See my calculation below.

Hamwi Equation

140 (My Ideal Body Weight)

x10

1,400 (Calories needed daily for BMR and to lose weight)

If my calories drop below 1,400 per day, I will lose significant lean-muscle mass because it's too low. An example of people whose calories significantly drop due to lack of consumed food and weight training are the homeless.

I've experienced something similar. When I was forty years young, I committed to keeping my weight between 145-150 lb. Then, I noticed it was fluctuating between 150 and 155 lb. I decided to lose five to ten pounds by eating less food and continued weight training. Within a couple months, however, a family member and I noticed that my quadriceps, hamstrings, buttocks, and abdominals weren't as lean and toned as before. I researched health and fitness resources and learned that I needed to consume a certain amount of calories daily in order to lose and/or maintain weight and functional-lean muscle mass.

I went back to eating my daily requirement of calories and gained weight and functional lean mass. Remember to eat the amount of calories you need for your daily BMR because if you eat more than needed, you risk gaining extra weight every year—especially if you're sedentary (inactive). For instance, if you eat 100 calories more than you need daily you'll gain about 10 pounds every year. Depending on your age and physical activity level that's an extra fifty pounds of weight in five years.

Men have a higher BMR requirement than women because they have more testosterone. For men to determine their Ideal Body Weight and BMR calories, they should use the following calculation.

For the first five feet of height, write 106 pounds. For each additional inch after five feet, multiply it by six. Add them up to determine your Ideal Body Weight. Then multiply it times ten to determine total calories needed daily at rest for BMR. For example, a man who is five feet eleven inches in height will have an Ideal Body Weight about 172 pounds. He needs about 1,720 calories per day for BMR.

As your body temple ages, it loses lean-muscle mass and metabolic rate decreases. However, with the Firm-Body Temple training program, you'll speed up your metabolic rate as you build lean-muscle mass and burn more calories while at rest or doing nothing. For example, you'll burn about sixty calories per hour instead of forty calories while you sleep. In a day, you'd burn an extra 540 calories while sleeping for nine hours. In about a week and with nine hours of sleep daily, your body would burn about 3,780 calories and lost about a pound of body fat.

It's beneficial that you lift weights or perform resistance training to build and maintain lean-muscle mass, rev up or increase your basal metabolic rate, and have a firm-body temple.

As our body temple ages, its metabolic rate decreases. In most people, it may cause an increase in body fat and a miserable quality of life—especially for the obese and elderly. This is especially challenging for many people who don't understand why they have difficulty losing weight (though they perform aerobic activities), getting up out of a chair or bed, and are losing lean-muscle mass.

We lose three percent of our muscle mass per decade. This is called sarcopenia. However, this isn't a result of aging, or only dieting. You'll need to perform strength or weight training to prevent this from happening to you.

In most of the USA and Europe, having a skinny or slim-body temple is coveted. Many skinny bodies have high percentage of body fat and may be deceiving, as a result. Sometimes the body is considered clinically or metabolically obese because it's weak. For example, I've observed many skinny or slim men and women rock backward to get up out of a chair. I've also seen people thrust their head forward to rise up out of their car seat. Why does this occur? They've lost significant functional-lean-muscle mass and strength.

Sarcopenia is also called "muscle wasting" by Barry Stein of Wake Forest University Medical School. Since muscle burns more energy than fat this means that metabolic load goes down and your metabolism reflects that. For example, if you're age eighty, sarcopenia started at age thirty. If you did no weight training, you've lost or wasted about fifteen percent of your lean-muscle mass.

Think of your muscles as your calorie-burning engine. If you're not strengthening your muscles with weight training, you're losing, neglecting, and weakening your engine. The good news is, when you perform the weight lifting exercises in this book, you can reduce your risk of losing and wasting your lean-muscle mass and gaining too much weight.

To burn calories and lose about a pound of body fat, you'll need to burn 3,500 calories. You can achieve this by walking, jogging, running, golfing, gardening or other purposeful, physical activities that you enjoy—about four to sixty minutes per day, minimum of two to four days per week. Perform weight training afterwards. I recommend aerobic and strength-weight training, two to four days per week.

The most common aerobic activity to burn excess calories is walking. If able, walking briskly is better. Some common rewards of walking are cardiovascular health, weight loss, functional, lean-muscle mass gain, disease and health ailments reduction, and happiness.

In general, you'll burn about 100 calories per mile walked or about 100 calories per 2,000 steps. Most public health agencies recommend walking 10,000 steps (five miles) per day to improve your health. Hence, if you walked five miles or 10,000 steps per day, you'll burn 500 calories. If you walked for seven days, you'll walk thirty-five miles or 70,000 steps and burn about 3,500 calories and lose one pound of body fat—in a week. It benefits your body temple to do physical activity like walking. Start walking and/or walk more today.

I was curious about calories burned if I walked instead of jog. I completed a personal *prevention trial* by walking thirty minutes per day instead of my usual light-moderate jogging. I wanted to see how many miles I could perform. When I jog, it takes about three minutes per lap and a total of 3.5 miles on a 400 m track.

The result of the trial illustrated that when I walked at a conversational pace (not briskly) or that of the average walker, I averaged about six minutes per lap and completed about a mile and a half. When comparing the walking results with the jogging results, the thirty-minute-prevention trial illustrated that I burned about half the calories while walking compared to jogging—about 150 calories with walking and 300 calories with jogging when performed with the same amount of time. In order for me to burn the same amount of calories when I jog, I must double my walking time and walk for sixty minutes instead.

Use my results to develop your own walking program to suit your calorie burning needs no matter what your fitness level. Walking isn't enough if your goal is to build a firm-body temple. You'll need to perform weight training after walking and stretching (2-4 days per week).

REV UP YOUR BMR

No matter what your fitness level, if you're able to move your body temple, you can rev up or increase your metabolic rate with exercise and functional-lean muscle mass through strength, weight or resistance training.

PERCENTAGE TO REV UP YOUR BMR DEPENDS ON FITNESS LEVEL

Sedentary (inactive, no exercise) - 30%

Work a job or moderately active – 50%

Work physically active job – 50%

Athletic (highly physically active) – 100%

For example: if I have a physically active job (waiter and waitress) and I'm getting regular exercise (both walking briskly and weight training), then I can double my daily **BMR** requirement from 1,400 calories to 2,800 calories. See calculation below.

<u>Hamwi Equation</u>

140 My Ideal Body Weight

<u>x10</u>

1,400 Calories I need daily for **BMR** (Basal Metabolic Rate) and to lose weight

<u>+1,400</u> Calories

2,800 Calories needed daily for my **BMR** and to lose weight

As a result, I can eat more food without worrying about increasing my body fat or gaining weight. I love to eat! This is one of the reasons I've been running and lifting weights after the Olympics.

2. THERMIC EFFECT OF FOOD

Another source of calorie burning is called Thermic Effect of Food. This is valuable information that many people don't know. This method uses calories to digest our foods. For example if you consume a protein meal, it's going to give you a thermic effect of food of about twenty-five of the meal's total calories. However, this isn't really practical because many of us aren't going to eat protein only meals-unless we're on one of those fad diets. The good news is if you want to really increase your calories needed to digest your meals, you must exercise.

The thermic effect of food increases your total energy expenditure between ten to thirty percent. However, when most people exercise after eating a meal, they increase the thermic effect of food from twenty to fifty six percent. That's amazing! The exception is with obese people.

After eating a meal, it's to your benefit to exercise. Rather, if you've eaten a large meal, you probably won't feel like exercising (jogging or running) afterward. Instead, you should walk a mile or two because you'll burn 100 calories per mile walked and significantly increase the calories needed to digest your meal.

For sedentary (inactive) and obese people enhancing the thermic effect of food may be challenging, but may be one of the solutions to solving weight management problems. So, use the Hamwi Equation to figure out your required energy intake and expenditure (output). For example, if you're obese and or sedentary, it's to your health benefit to walk in place while talking on the telephone and watching television, park in the farthest row of the supermarket, mall, spiritual center, your job or business parking lot. Walk in the parking lot or around the block on your break times.

Former First Lady Michelle Obama's health campaign (*Lets' Move!)* was developed to solve the childhood obesity epidemic. Similarly, both *Irresistibly Fit* and my exercise, *Althea*, were created to solve the global childhood and adult obesity and depression epidemic. So, use my resources. Many people in the world have told me that they work for them.

3. PHYSICAL ACTIVITY LEVEL

Another source of calorie burning is physical activity or exercise. It's amazing and significant because it accounts for fifteen to thirty percent of your total energy expenditure. If you're sedentary, you're missing out on this amazing benefit. However, if you're physically active and exercising, you're benefiting in many ways. For example, if I'm exercising with aerobic and weight training exercises, I'll increase my total energy expenditure about thirty percent. That means I can add thirty percent more calories to my BMR (1,400 calories). See the calculation below.

Hamwi Equation

140 My Ideal Body Weight

x10

1,400 Calories needed daily for my BMR (Basal Metabolic Rate) and to lose weight

+ 420 Calories (30% of 1,400)

1,820 Calories needed daily for my BMR and to lose weight

This absolutely excites me because it allows me to eat more food without gaining excess fat or weight—as long as I'm physically active two to four days per week.

Physical activity is necessary for building a firm-body temple and having optimal health. It's necessary to burn the maximum amount of calories, lose fat and water (weight) and toxins, strengthen muscles, and decrease the risk of degenerative diseases and conditions (heart, diabetes, high blood pressure, cholesterol, and gout). Exercise makes us feel happy or happier due to flowing chemicals (endorphins) in our brain.

Weight training promotes functional-lean-muscle mass much more than walking and other aerobic activities. It's likely to prevent you from out-eating or out-drinking your aerobic exercise.

I've found that many people, who only do average aerobic and/or no weight-training activities overestimate its value. Many times they out-eat or out-drink their exercise the same day. If they walked five miles, they burned about 500 calories. However, if they ate a poppyseed muffin with 500 calories, they out-ate their exercise.

Even so, if after walking three and a half miles and burning 350 calories someone ate an apple bran muffin with 350 calories, they out-ate their exercise. If they drank a margarita after walking six miles and burning 600 calories, they out-drank their exercise. On the other hand, if they weight trained after the aerobic exercise, it's unlikely they'd out-eat their exercise.

In summary, your total energy expenditure is determined by three sources that influence your muscle mass or calorie burning engine at these rates. Knowing this gives you a better chance to be irresistibly fit forever.

Total Energy Expenditure determined by:

Percentage accounted for

Basal Metabolic Rate (unit of energy burned)	60-75%
Thermic Effect of Food (calories burned for digestion)	10-30%
Physical Activity Level (calories burned when exercising)	15-30%

How will you sustain your physical activity level? I enjoy light jogging, so I jog. I also enjoy my technique *ALTHEA*, HIIT or High Intensity Interval Training, bike riding, and lifting weights. You should perform the activities that you enjoy the most. If you enjoy running, run. If you enjoy bike riding, ride. If you enjoy gardening, do gardening. If you enjoy golfing, golf. Don't forget to perform strength and weight training techniques from this book because the more functional-lean-muscle mass you build the more calories you'll burn.

THREE IMPORTANT NUTRIENTS

Your body needs a complete balance of healthy nutrients (macronutrients and micronutrients) to function properly. Micronutrients clean, nourish and help your cells resist diseases. Macronutrients are carbohydrates, protein, and fats. Micronutrients are vitamins, minerals, and healthy water.

Recent studies show Americans are consuming about sixty percent of macronutrients from processed foods and thirty percent from meats, and only five percent nutrients from grains, nuts, and seeds, and five percent from fruits and vegetables. It's important to be conscious of the functions and benefits of these essential nutrients to make healthy nutritional food and water choices for optimal health and a fit body temple.

CARBOHYDRATES

In the early 1900s, people ate many carbohydrates by way of whole foods, like grains, fruits, and vegetables—but it didn't lead to a health epidemic. However, in this new millennium, carbohydrates have been getting a bad rap due to weight gain. Carbohydrates aren't all bad for you. Carbohydrate's primary function is to produce usable energy. They're made up of carbon, hydrogen, and oxygen. It's our body's main source of fuel for energy.

Studies show when carbohydrates are digested, they're converted into glucose or blood sugar—the excess is stored in your liver and muscles for future use. It's the exclusive fuel source that keeps our central nervous system and brain functioning properly.

PROTEIN

Protein is an indispensable nutrient—the basic building block for building, repairing, and maintaining tissues in the body. Protein is found in every cell and tissue in our body—especially muscles. It's in your fingernails, hair, blood, internal organs, and bones.

Protein ignites your fat burning hormones. It's responsible for building strong bones during childhood and important for maintaining bone mass as we age. It may help reverse bone loss as we age too.

Protein is broken down in your stomach and intestines. It's made up of twenty-one amino acids—essential and non-essential. The body doesn't make essential proteins, so you need to consume foods to obtain them. You can eat complete protein foods (all meats, poultry, fish, dairy, and eggs) because they contain all the essential proteins you need. Also, soy products contain all the essential proteins needed and are the only complete protein for vegetarians. Non-essential proteins are made by the body under normal circumstances.

Furthermore, the body doesn't store protein like it does fat. You'll need to replenish protein daily, or you may experience loss of function in your muscles, liver, and white blood cells.

You can eat complementary protein foods because they provide both essential and non-essential proteins. Example: beans and rice, wheat bread and peanut butter sandwich. In the past, studies suggested you needed to eat them together to get the protein, but new studies show you don't. You must eat them in the same day.

Protein can be found in a variety of foods like meats, poultry, fish, eggs, tofu, legumes, nuts and seeds, milk and milk products, grains, and some fruits and vegetables. However, fruits and vegetables provide a small amount of protein. Thus, it's important to check food ingredients and what your body needs to make healthy choices.

If you're physically active, and performing strength or weight training, and or managing your weight, you need a balanced intake of high-protein and low-calorie foods.

Protein intake requirements for the physically active and athletes are debated considerably. But, everyone can benefit from protein intake. Your protein requirement is mostly determined by your overall energy and carbohydrates intake, need for essential proteins, body weight and composition, rate of physical activity level, and injury or illness.

Studies show that weight-training athletes need more protein than physically active and endurance athletes, and physically active and endurance athletes need more than normal sedentary adults. Since more protein is lost, more protein is beneficial for both active groups—active and endurance athletes break down muscles and weight training athletes tear muscles when building them, and have bigger muscle mass. There's also sweat loss and energy expenditure resulting in the need for more energy and repairing of muscles.

The best sources of high protein foods are seafood and poultry because they're high in protein with low calorie counts. This is essential because protein intake contributes to your calorie intake. If you consume too much protein and calories, it can increase weight gain and or lead to obesity, which leads to chronic diseases and no firm-body temple.

I don't recommend red meat for protein because they're high in fat, takes about three days to digest, linked to colorectal cancers, and the heme iron is easily absorbed in your body and linked to heart attacks and heart disease.

A study by Harvard School of Public Health revealed that red meat consumption was associated with a higher risk of early death due to the red meats participants in the study reported they ate. They were more likely to die during the twenty-year time the data was collected. Consume less red meat and remove excess fat and skins from seafood and poultry.

Protein has four calories per gram, like carbohydrates. If you consume forty grams of protein, you've consumed about 160 calories. NOTE: If you don't eat red meat, poultry or fish, you should consume a combination of beans and rice, and other complementary-protein foods or supplements to get the protein needed.

WATER

Water is an essential nutrient for your body and life. Your body is made up of sixty to seventy-five percent water. It's your transportation system that moves nutrients, fat, and toxins from your trillions of cells, and waste material from your body. It lubricates your brain, eyes, spinal chords, and joints.

Water aids in biochemical reactions by assisting digestion of proteins and carbohydrates. Your body has an intricate system that works to help with water balance. Water regulates your body temperature by slowly changing the temperature and serving as a good heat storage substance for it. Evaporation of water from your skin surface helps to cool your body. More than two quarts of water is lost from a typical adult's body (about 3/4 through urine) and more from those who exercise.

Other water losses are from sweat, tiny droplets of air from breathing, energy metabolism, and feces. It's essential that your water losses are replaced and balanced with your daily water intake—it helps to prevent dehydration.

I recommend drinking fifty percent of your body weight in ounces. For example, if your body weight is 120 lb, divide it by fifty percent. That's sixty pounds. Change pounds to ounces. Divide sixty pounds by eight cups. That's seven and a half cups. A 120 lb person needs about seven and a half cups of water daily.

Start today with a plan and the information in this book to become irresistibly fit. To your success, happiness, longevity, good quality of life, and wellness.

If you do not change direction you may end up where you were heading. -Lao Tzu

APPENDIX

ALARMING-GLOBAL HEALTH STATISTICS

70% American adults are overweight or obese (2013-2014) CDC

More than 300 million people are obese across the world

Around 1 billion people are estimated to be overweight across the globe.

Cardiovascular disease is the leading cause of death globally. (WHO atlas)

Heart disease kills 7.1 million people/year globally. (2013)

630,000 (1 in 4 deaths) Americans die of heart disease per year. (2017) (CDC)

Physical inactivity and unhealthy diet are other main risk factors that increase individual risk of cardiovascular diseases. (WHO Atlas)

70% diseases are caused by our lifestyle choices.

BENEFITS OF PROTEIN

Helps you:

- Look better
- Build new and maintain muscle
- Lose fat

Important:

- Complete protein is from animal sources
- Mainly incomplete protein is from vegetable sources
- Essential means your body can't manufacture that amino acid

Example: Beans and brown rice together are complete proteins

HIGH PROTEIN FOODS LIST

This list of high protein foods has only seafood and poultry. Because they're such high protein sources with low calorie counts, I love to consume them without guilt. The lean poultry and fish are at the top of the healthy list for best sources of protein.

SEAFOOD - protein and carbohydrates listed in grams

High Protein Sources	Serving	Protein	Carbs	Calories
Anchovies, in water	1 ounce	6	0	37
Crab, king (cooked)	4 ounces	22	0	110
Flounder & Sole (cooked)	4 ounces	27	0	133
Haddock (baked or broiled)	4 ounces	28	0	127
Herring (cooked)	4 ounces	26	0	230
Mahi Mahi (baked or broiled)	4 ounces	27	0	124
Perch (freshwater) (cooked)	4 ounces	28	0	133
Pollock (baked or broiled	4 ounces	28	0	134

Salmon (baked or broiled)	4 ounces	25	0	234
Sardines, in water	1 can	22	0	130
Scallops (steamed)	4 ounces	26	0	127
Shrimp	4 ounces	24	0	112
Snapper (baked or broiled)	4 ounces	30	0	145
Trout, freshwater (cooked)	4 ounces	30	0	215
Tuna, canned (chunk lite)	1/4 cup	16	0	70
Whitefish (baked or broiled)	4 ounces	28	0	195

*Avoid high-mercury shark, swordfish, king mackerel, marlin and tilefish.

POULTRY - protein and carbohydrates listed in grams

High Protein Sources	Serving	Protein	Carbs	Calories
Chicken breast	4 ounces	29	0	193
Chicken, light meat (no skin)	4 ounces	35	0	196
Chicken, dark meat (no skin)	4 ounces	31	0	232
Turkey, light meat (no skin)	4 ounces	34	0	178
Turkey, dark meat (no skin)	4 ounces	32	0	212

The "B" High Protein Foods List

The "B" list of high protein foods contains dairy and legumes (beans, peas and lentils). Dairy is also important for calcium. And beans, peas and lentils are your best sources of protein from high fiber plant foods.

DAIRY - protein and carbohydrates listed in grams

High Protein Sources	Serving	Protein	Carbs	Calories
Cheddar cheese	1 ounce	7	<1	114

Cheddar, low-fat	1 ounce	8	1	90
Cottage cheese	1/2 cup	14	3	110
Cottage cheese, low-fat	1/2 cup	16	3	90
Egg	1 large	6	0	75
Milk, low-fat	1 cup	8	12	121
Milk, skim	1 cup	8	12	86
Muenster cheese	1 ounce	7	<1	104
Swiss cheese	1 ounce	8	1	107
Yogurt, low-fat	1 cup	12	16	144
Yogurt, nonfat	1 cup	13	17	127

LEGUMES - protein and carbohydrates listed in grams

High Protein Sources	Serving	Protein	Carbs	Calories
Black beans (cooked)	1/2 cup	8	20	113
Garbanzo/chickpeas (cooked)	1/2 cup	7	23	134
Kidney beans (cooked)	1/2 cup	8	20	112
Lentil beans (cooked)	1/2 cup	9	20	115
Lima beans (cooked)	1/2 cup	7	20	108
Navy beans (cooked)	1/2 cup	8	24	129
Soybeans/edamame (cooked)	1/2 cup	11	10	127
Tofu (fresh)	1/2 cup	10	2	94

The "C" High Protein Foods List

Even though whole grains and nuts are on the "C" list of high protein foods, they're both loaded with fiber and nutrition. And when combined with legumes, the combination boosts your total healthy protein intake.

GRAINS - protein and carbohydrates listed in grams

High Protein Sources	Serving	Protein	Carbs	Calories
Oatmeal, rolled oats (cooked)	1 cup	6	25	145
Pancake, buckwheat	1 4"	2	6	54
Pancake, whole wheat	1 4"	3	9	74
Pasta, whole wheat (cooked)	1 cup	7	37	174
Popcorn, dry (cooked)	1 cup	2	11	54
Rice, brown (cooked)	1/2 cup	2	23	108
Rye bread	1 slice	2	12	56
Whole wheat bread	1 slice	2	11	56

NUTS - protein and carbohydrates listed in grams

High Protein Sources	Serving	Protein	Carbs	Calories
Almonds (23 nuts)	1 ounce	6	6	162
Brazil nuts	1 ounce	4	3	184
Cashews	1 ounce	4	9	155
Filberts (hazelnuts)	1 ounce	4	5	176
Peanuts	1 ounce	8	4	168
Peanut butter	2 Tabs.	8	6	188
Pecans	1 ounce	3	4	193
Pistachios	1 ounce	6	8	160
Walnuts	1 ounce	4	4	185

(Anonymous source)

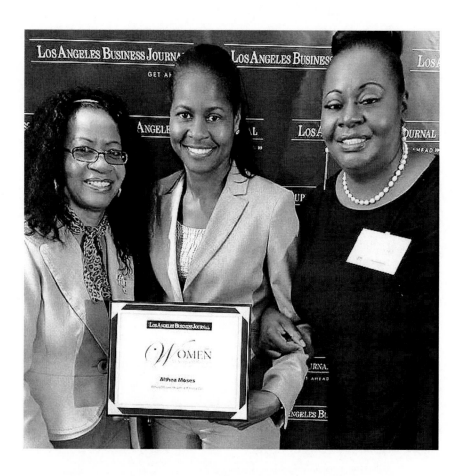

Women Making A Difference Nominee Award
(Los Angeles Business Journal)

More about Althea Moses

- Wrote first book, *IRRESISTIBLY FIT* (2013)
- **Published Author** on Ezinearticles.com
- **Founded Althea Moses Health & Fitness Co.** (2013)
- **Created ALTHEA**: an innovative mind/body exercise
- **Invented the Circlemark** Circle Hand Gesture
- Designs world-class health & fitness programs that work in little time
- **Produced and hosted weekly radio show**: HOT Health & Fitness Tips With The Olympian, Althea Moses (2014 - 2016)
- **Los Angeles Business Journal**, Women Making A Difference nominated for Rising Star Award (2014 and 2015)
- Launched **Althea Moses Health & Fitness Co.** (2014)
- Launched **ALTHEA group fitness classes** in Los Angeles (2014)
- Launched **ALTHEA Fitness studio** in Los Angeles (2014)
- Special Guest Trainer - **Playa Vista Certified Farmers Market** in Playa Vista (2014 and 2015)
- Special Guest Trainer - **Motor Avenue Farmers Market** in Los Angeles (2014)
- Special Guest Trainer at Annual **LAUSD 5K** Move It Challenge & Health Fair (2014 - 2016)
- Special Guest Trainer at Annual **Girl Scouts** "Family Fit Fair" (2014 and 2015)
- Special Guest on **A Taste of Belize TV Show** with Host Sandra Gillett (2014)
- Special Guest on **Morning Matters TV Show** with Rhonda Crichton (2015)

- City of Inglewood **Ambassador** for Host Town Activities - **Special Olympic World Games** in Los Angeles (2015)
- Launched **Althea Moses Fitness Club** at Edward Vincent, Jr. Park in Inglewood (2015)
- **City of Inglewood Grand Marshal** for MLK, Jr. Day Celebration - Presented keynote speech (2016)
- Launched **ALTHEA group fitness class** at Darby Park Studio in Inglewood - near future Rams stadium (2016)
- **Los Angeles Business Journal,** Women's Summit nominated Rising Star Award (2016 and 2017)
- Featured in the **VoyageLA magazine** (2017)
- Published first book, ***IRRESISTIBLY FIT*** - It became a #1 bestseller in 24 hours and international bestseller in three days on Amazon.com
- **#1 International - Bestselling Author** (2017, 2018)

TESTIMONIALS:
www.Linkedin.com
(https://www.linkedin.com/pub/althea-moses/16/490/699)

www.altheam.com

HOW TO BOOK & CONTACT ALTHEA

Book Althea Moses for consultations, speaking events, fitness performance events, interviews, talk shows or reality television shows. Hire Althea Moses as your keynote speaker. We guarantee that your event will be educational, entertaining, and unforgettable.

Contact: **info@altheam.com**

Website: **ALTHEAM.COM**

Radio Talk Show: Hot Health & Fitness Tips on www.blogtalkradio.com/altheamoses

Follow on Social Media:

Althea Moses on www.instagram.com (https://instagram.com/altheamoses)

Althea Moses on www.facebook.com (https://www.facebook.com/altheamosesolympian)

Althea Moses Health and Fitness Co. on www.facebook.com (https://www.facebook.com/altheamoseshealthandfitness)

Althea Moses on www.linkedin.com (https://www.linkedin.com/in/althea-moses-69949016/)

Althea Moses on www.twitter.com (https://twitter.com/altheamoses)

Althea Moses Health & Fitness Co. on www.twitter.com (https://twitter.com/altheamosesheal)

Althea Moses YouTube Channel www.youtube.com (www.youtube.com/user/1996olympian)

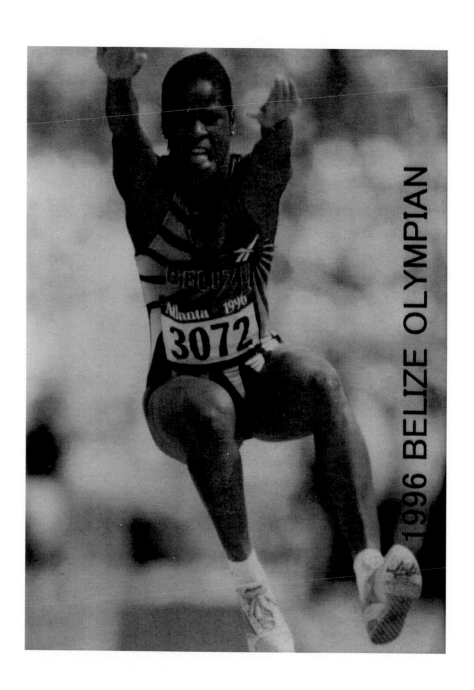

1996 BELIZE OLYMPIAN

About the Author

Althea Moses is a Belizean #1 international, bestselling author, Olympian, consultant, personal coach, speaker, creator, advisor, lead-group-fitness trainer, boss lady of fitness. She was raised in Belize before immigrating to Los Angeles and Inglewood, California.

Althea became a silver medalist in the 1986 Jr. Olympics, an Olympic record-breaking-gold medalist in 1987, graduated from UCLA in 1993, and competed in the 1996 Olympic Games in Atlanta, Georgia. In 2001, she earned a Masters degree in Education and California Teaching Credential. She taught elementary school for eleven years -- she was laid off in 2009.

She is the former fiancé of the legendary-music producer, singer, songwriter, author, and humanitarian, Kashif Saleem.

In 2013, she founded Althea Moses Health and Fitness Co., created the exercise, (ALTHEA), invented the Circlemark, and wrote her first book, Irresistibly Fit, in Los Angeles, California.

She is a fitness model.

For more than four years, she has been a personal coach for many women in greater Los Angeles, California. The Office of former First Lady Michelle Obama recognized ALTHEA (exercise) in 2015. She was an active Let's Move! trainer in greater Los Angeles.

In 2014 and 2015, and 2016, Althea was nominated for a Los Angeles Business Journal's Women Making A Difference Award.

In 2014, Althea launched, produced, and hosted weekly radio show, HOT Health & Fitness Tips on Blogtalkradio.com She produced 90 episodes in two years.

Althea launched and operates the ALTHEA group fitness classes in Los Angeles and Inglewood. In 2015, she founded and volunteers for the Althea Moses Fitness Club--a free fitness program for the residents of Inglewood and greater Los Angeles.

In 2016, Althea was a Grand marshal of the City of Inglewood's Dr. Martin Luther King, Jr. Day Celebration. In 2017, she was featured in VoyageLA magazine and nominated for a Los Angeles Business Journal's Women's Summit award.

In December 2017, Althea published her first book, *Irresistibly Fit*. It teaches women how to combine spiritual and physical exercises to become strong, firm, and sexy in little time. Her book debuted as a #1 bestseller in the US (in 1 day), and the United Kingdom, Canada, and Australia (in three days).

In 2018, LAUSD educators recognized Althea Moses as an African-American Achiever during Black History Month.

In 2018, the City of Inglewood awarded Althea for her volunteer service--Althea Moses Fitness Club.

Althea resides in Inglewood and Los Angeles, California.

Thank you for purchasing my book. If the information added value to your life, please write your Review on Amazon by going to these links

https://www.facebook.com/altheamoseshealthandfitness/

and

www.amazon.com

Please don't keep me a secret. If you received value from my book, trainings or programs, please introduce me to someone you know, who could benefit also—Register at www.altheam.com/contact or email info@altheam.com

Thank you for your support! I appreciate you!

ALTHEA'S FREE NEWSLETTER

Get expert tips, offers, free downloads, and evites to special events delivered to your inbox.

We promise never to sell or rent your email address.

Click this link www.altheam.com to register today.